S0-APQ-777

Clinical Pocket Manual™

Neurologic Care

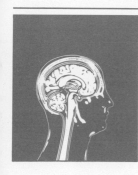

NURSING87 BOOKS™
SPRINGHOUSE CORPORATION
SPRINGHOUSE, PENNSYLVANIA

Clinical Pocket Manual™ Series

PROGRAM DIRECTOR
Jean Robinson

CLINICAL DIRECTOR
Barbara McVan, RN

ART DIRECTOR
John Hubbard

EDITORIAL MANAGER
Susan R. Williams

EDITORS
Lisa Z. Cohen
Kathy E. Goldberg
Virginia P. Peck

CLINICAL EDITORS
Donna Hilton, RN, CCRN, CEN
Joan E. Mason, RN, EdM
Diane Schweisguth, RN, BSN

EDITORIAL SERVICES
SUPERVISOR
David R. Moreau

DESIGNER
Maria Errico

PRODUCTION COORDINATOR
Susan Powell-Mishler

Material in this book was adapted from the following series: Nurse's Reference Library, Nursing Photobook, New Nursing Skillbook, Nursing Now, and Nurse's Clinical Library.

Amended reprint, 1987

Library of Congress Cataloging-in-Publication Data

Main entry under title:

Neurologic care.

(Clinical pocket manual)
"Nursing86 books."
Includes index.
1. Neurological nursing—Handbooks, manuals, etc.
2. Nervous system—Diseases—Handbooks, manuals, etc.   I. Series. [DNLM: 1. Neurology—handbooks. WL 39 N494]
RC350.5.N467   1986   616.8   85-27706
ISBN 0-87434-011-X

CONTENTS

Nursing87 Books™

CLINICAL POCKET MANUAL™ SERIES

Diagnostic Tests
Emergency Care
Fluids and Electrolytes
Signs and Symptoms
Cardiovascular Care
Respiratory Care
Critical Care
Neurologic Care
Surgical Care
Medications and I.V.s
Ob/Gyn Care
Pediatric Care

NURSING NOW™ SERIES

Shock
Hypertension
Drug Interactions
Cardiac Crises
Respiratory Emergencies
Pain

NURSE'S CLINICAL LIBRARY®

Cardiovascular Disorders
Respiratory Disorders
Endocrine Disorders
Neurologic Disorders
Renal and Urologic Disorders
Gastrointestinal Disorders
Neoplastic Disorders
Immune Disorders

NURSE'S REFERENCE LIBRARY®

Diseases	Definitions
Diagnostics	Practices
Drugs	Emergencies
Assessment	Signs & Symptoms
Procedures	Patient Teaching

NURSING PHOTOBOOK™ SERIES

Providing Respiratory Care
Managing I.V. Therapy
Dealing with Emergencies
Giving Medications
Assessing Your Patients
Using Monitors
Providing Early Mobility
Giving Cardiac Care
Performing GI Procedures
Implementing Urologic Procedures
Controlling Infection
Ensuring Intensive Care
Coping with Neurologic Disorders
Caring for Surgical Patients
Working with Orthopedic Patients
Nursing Pediatric Patients
Helping Geriatric Patients
Attending Ob/Gyn Patients
Aiding Ambulatory Patients
Carrying Out Special Procedures

NURSE REVIEW™ SERIES

Cardiac Problems
Respiratory Problems
Gastrointestinal Problems
Neurologic Problems
Vascular Problems
Genitourinary Problems
Endocrine Problems
Musculoskeletal Problems

Nursing87 DRUG HANDBOOK™

Assessing Your Patient's Level of Consciousness Using the Glasgow Coma Scale

To assess and monitor the level of consciousness of a patient with suspected or confirmed brain injury, use the Glasgow Coma Scale. You'll find this scale useful in the emergency department, at the scene of an accident, and for vital assessment of the hospitalized patient. The Glasgow Scale measures three faculties' responses to stimuli—*eye opening*, *motor response*, and *verbal response*. Below you'll find an expanded version of this useful—though not comprehensive—assessment technique. (The lowest a patient can score is 3, the highest 15. A patient scoring 7 or less is comatose and probably has severe neurologic damage.)

TEST	SCORE	PATIENT'S RESPONSE
Verbal response (when you ask, "What year is this?")		
Oriented	5	He tells you the current year.
Confused	4	He telis you an incorrect year.
Inappropriate words	3	He replies randomly: "tomorrow" or "roses."
Incomprehensible	2	He moans or screams.
None	1	He gives no response.
Eye opening response		
Spontaneously	4	He opens his eyes spontaneously.
To speech	3	He opens his eyes when you tell him to.
To pain	2	He opens his eyes only on painful stimulus (for example, application of pressure to bony ridge under eyebrow).
None	1	He doesn't open his eyes in response to any stimulus.

Continued

Assessing Your Patient's Level of Consciousness Using the Glasgow Coma Scale
Continued

TEST	SCORE	PATIENT'S RESPONSE
Motor Response		
Obeys	6	He shows you two fingers when you ask him to.
Localizes	5	He reaches toward the painful stimulus and tries to remove it.
Withdraws	4	He moves away from a painful stimulus.
Abnormal flexion	3	He assumes a decorticate posture (below).

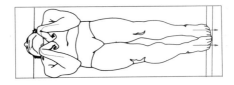

Abnormal extension	2	He assumes a decerebrate posture (below).

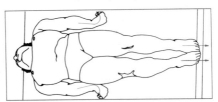

None	1	He doesn't respond at all, just lies flaccid—an *ominous sign*.

Neurologic Check

The chart below shows the changes in mental state, pupil dilation, and vital signs that accompany a fatal increase of intracranial pressure.

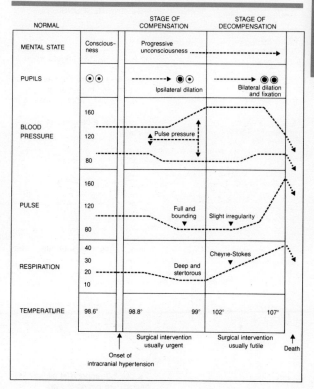

PATIENT EVALUATION

Assessing Respiratory Function

In an unconscious patient, these patterns of respiration indicate neurologic abnormalities.

PATTERN OF RESPIRATION	CHARACTERISTICS	SIGNIFICANCE
Cheyne-Stokes	• Rhythmic waxing and waning of both rate and depth of respirations, alternating regularly with briefer periods of apnea	• May indicate deep cerebral or cerebellar lesions, usually bilateral; may occur with upper brain stem involvement
Central neurogenic hyperventilation	• Sustained, regular, rapid respirations with forced inspiration and expiration	• May indicate a lesion of the low midbrain or upper pons areas of the brain stem
Apneustic	• Prolonged inspiratory cramp with a pause at full inspiration; there may also be expiratory pauses	• May indicate a lesion of the mid- or low pons
Cluster breathing	• Clusters of irregular respirations alternating with longer periods of apnea	• May indicate a lesion of the low pons or upper medulla
Ataxic breathing	• A completely irregular pattern with random deep and shallow respirations; irregular pauses may also appear	• May indicate a lesion of the medulla

Visual Field Check

Perform this simple test if you suspect your patient has a neurologic problem affecting his peripheral vision. If results suggest a visual defect, his doctor may wish to perform a more detailed exam using special techniques.

Here's how you do it: First, position yourself so you're facing the patient, eyes level with his, about 2 feet away. Then, ask him to cover one eye without pressing on it, and to look at your eye directly opposite. Bring a pencil or another small object from the periphery into his field of vision. Do this from several directions, as illustrated. Each time, ask him to indicate when he first sees the object coming into view, and compare the extent of his vision with yours. Then repeat the test with his other eye.

Note: To test the medial field, keep the test object equidistant between you and the patient. To test the lateral field, start with the object somewhat behind the patient.

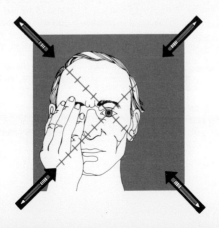

PATIENT EVALUATION

Grading Pupils

Monitoring your patient's pupillary activity is an important part of neurologic nursing care. But how do you compare your findings at, say, 4 p.m. with those of another nurse at 2 p.m.? To do so, you need to know something more specific than "right pupil more dilated than left."

To help you and other health-team members compare findings, here's a way to evaluate pupil sizes precisely: Put a scale showing sizes in millimeters at the top of the patient's flow chart. Then, each nurse can compare pupillary changes against an absolute, and identical, frame of reference.

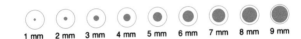

1 mm   2 mm   3 mm   4 mm   5 mm   6 mm   7 mm   8 mm   9 mm

Interpreting Your Findings

Now that you've tested your patient's pupillary reflexes, how do you interpret your findings? Watch for a sluggish reaction to light and report it promptly. In many cases, it's an early warning that the patient's condition is deteriorating. Unequal pupil sizes may indicate his parasympathetic

and sympathetic nervous systems aren't working together as they should. If your patient has a dilated and nonreactive pupil on only one side, *call the doctor immediately*. This could be from increased intracranial pressure, or ipsilateral oculomotor nerve compression from tumor or injury.

Oculocephalic Reflex

How can you quickly assess brain stem function in an unconscious patient? Test his oculocephalic reflex, which is sometimes called doll's eye reflex. To test for this reflex, hold the patient's eyelids open. Then, quickly—but gently—turn his head to the right. If everything's OK, his eyes will appear to move conjugately toward the center of his body (left of his eye sockets). But if his eyes remain stationary in the center or to the right of his eye sockets, his doll's eye reflex is absent, indicating a deteriorating consciousness level. Notify the doctor.

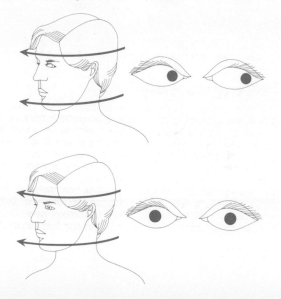

Identifying Dermatomes

To document your patient's sensory function, you'll use a body chart, like the one shown here, illustrating cutaneous nerve distribution. The left half of this figure shows the distribution of spinal nerves; the right half shows the distribution of cutaneous fields of peripheral nerves.

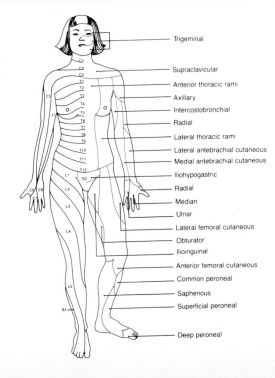

- Trigeminal
- Supraclavicular
- Anterior thoracic rami
- Axillary
- Intercostobronchial
- Radial
- Lateral thoracic rami
- Lateral antebrachial cutaneous
- Medial antebrachial cutaneous
- Iliohypogastric
- Radial
- Median
- Ulnar
- Lateral femoral cutaneous
- Obturator
- Ilioinguinal
- Anterior femoral cutaneous
- Common peroneal
- Saphenous
- Superficial peroneal
- Deep peroneal

Identifying Dermatomes
Continued

Here's an example of how to document the specific areas tested and the test results: Assume your patient can't feel a pinprick on her right index and middle fingers. Using the chart, you'd document this finding as a loss of pain sensation in the C7 area. Remember, you may find minor variations in the exact segmental levels, depending on the chart you're using.

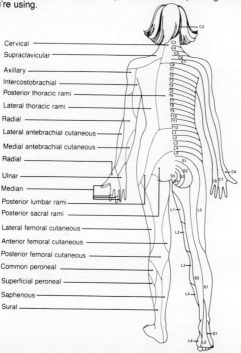

Cervical
Supraclavicular
Axillary
Intercostobrachial
Posterior thoracic rami
Lateral thoracic rami
Radial
Lateral antebrachial cutaneous
Medial antebrachial cutaneous
Radial
Ulnar
Median
Posterior lumbar rami
Posterior sacral rami
Lateral femoral cutaneous
Anterior femoral cutaneous
Posterior femoral cutaneous
Common peroneal
Superficial peroneal
Saphenous
Sural

PATIENT EVALUATION

Observing Your Patient's Gait

TYPE	CHARACTERISTICS	POSSIBLE DISORDER
Ataxic	Staggering; unsteadiness; inability to remain steady with feet together; tendency to reel to one side	Disease of the cerebellum or posterior columns
Dystonic	Irregular, nondirective movements	Disorder of muscle tone
Dystrophic	Waddling, with legs far apart; weight shifts from side to side; abdomen protrudes; lordosis possible	Weakness of pelvic girdle; dislocated hip
Hemiplegic	Rigid movements; leg on affected side circles outward, foot drags on floor, arm on same side may be rigidly flexed and does not swing freely; leaning to affected side	Disorder of corticospinal tract
Parkinsonian	Forward-leaning posture, head bent, hips and knees flexed; short, shuffled, rapidly accelerating steps; stiff turns, entire body rotated at once; difficulty starting and stopping	Basal ganglia defects of Parkinson's disease; extrapyramidal tract
Scissors	Short, slow steps, with legs alternately crossing over each other	Spastic paraplegia
Spastic	Short steps, dragging balls of feet	Bilateral lesion of corticospinal tract
Steppage	Exaggerated, high steps, with knees flexed; feet brought down heavily	Footdrop secondary to lower motor neuron lesions

Grading Reflexes

When testing your patient's deep tendon and superficial reflexes, use the following grading scales:

Deep tendon reflex grades
0 absent
1+ present but diminished
2+ normal
3+ increased but not necessarily pathologic
4+ hyperactive; clonus may also be present

Superficial reflex grades
0 absent
± equivocal or barely present
+ normally active

Record the patient's reflex scores by drawing a stick figure and entering the scores at the proper location. The figure shown here indicates normal deep tendon reflex activity as well as normal superficial reflex activity over the abdominal area. The arrows at the figure's feet indicate normal plantar reflex activity.

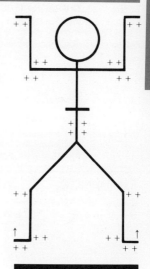

Plantar Reflex

Stroke the lateral aspect of the sole of your patient's foot (left). The normal response is flexion of the toes (center).

The Babinski response is abnormal. The great toe will dorsiflex and the other toes fan (right). This indicates an upper motor neuron lesion.

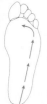
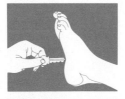
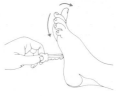

Patellar Reflex—"Knee Jerk"

Here's an example of a deep tendon reflex. To elicit this reflex when your patient's lying down, place your hand under his knee to raise and flex it.

Then tap his patellar tendon just below the knee with a reflex hammer. If he responds normally, his leg will extend.

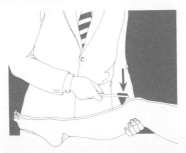

Other Common Deep Tendon Reflex Tests

The most commonly assessed deep tendon reflexes are as follows:

• *Biceps.* To elicit this reflex, have the patient relax his arm and pronate the forearm slightly, positioned somewhere between flexion and extension. (For best results, ask the patient to rest his elbow in your hand.) Then, percuss the biceps tendon with the reflex hammer. The biceps muscle should contract, followed by flexion of the forearm.

• *Brachioradialis.* Position the patient's forearm in semiflexion and semipronation, resting it either in your hand or on his knee. Tap the styloid process of the radius 1″ to 2″ (2.5 to 5 cm) above the wrist. You should see flexion at the elbow and a simultaneous pronation of the forearm, as well as flexion of the fingers and hand.

• *Triceps.* Position the patient's arm about midway between flexion and extension. If possible, have the patient rest his arm on his thigh or in your hand. Tap the tendon above the insertion on the ulna's olecranon process, 1″ to 2″ above the elbow. The stimulus should elicit muscle contraction of the triceps and elbow extension.

• *Achilles.* Have the patient sit on a table with his legs dangling. (If the patient can't sit without support, have him sit or lie in bed.) Flex his leg at the hip and knee, and rotate it externally. If the patient is prone, flex his knee and hip and rotate the leg externally so that it rests on the opposite shin. Then, place your hand under the patient's foot, dorsiflex the ankle, and tap the tendon just above its insertion on the posterior surface of the calcaneus. You should see a plantar flexion of the foot at the ankle.

Testing Muscle Strength

1. Place your patient's leg with knee flexed and foot resting on the bed, as shown here. Instruct him to keep his foot down as you try to extend his leg.

2. Support his knee as shown in the illustration. Instruct him to straighten his leg as you apply resistance.

Evaluate and document your patient's performance. Incorporate your assessment in his care plan.

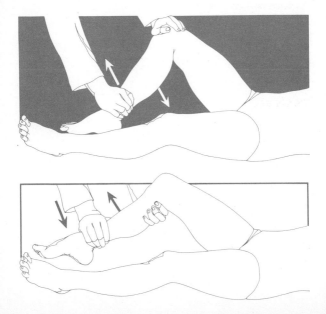

Rating Scale for Muscle Strength

Muscle tone and strength. Before assessing muscle tone or resistance to passive movement, encourage the patient to relax. Then move his joints through passive range of motion (ROM). Palpate the muscles for consistency, passive elasticity, and firmness as you do so. Note any muscle tenderness.

Next, assess muscle strength. Have the patient perform active ROM against your resistance (see *Testing muscle strength*, page 14).

To record the patient's muscle strength, use this rating scale:

5/5: Patient moves joint through full range of motion (ROM) against normal resistance and gravity.
4/5: Patient completes full ROM against moderate resistance and gravity.
3/5: Patient completes full ROM against gravity only.
2/5: Patient completes full ROM but not against gravity.
1/5: Patient's attempt at muscle contraction is palpable, but limb doesn't move.
0/5: Patient makes no visible or palpable muscle contraction; muscle is paralyzed.

Coordination

The following tests evaluate purposeful, fine movements and coordination of the arms and legs.

With the patient seated facing you, begin assessing his coordination by testing his arms. Ask him to touch each finger rapidly with his thumb, rhythmically pat his leg with his hand, and quickly turn his hand over and back. Have the patient perform each maneuver with each hand for about 30 seconds. Then, ask him to touch your index finger, then his nose, several times. Have him repeat this maneuver with his eyes closed.

To test leg coordination, ask the patient to tap his foot on the floor or on your palm. Then ask him to place the heel of one foot on his other knee and slide the heel down his shin.

As the patient performs all these tests, observe for slowness, tremor, or awkwardness.

Guide to Cranial Nerve Assessment

Thorough neurologic examination includes assessment of the 12 cranial nerves, which may have sensory or motor functions, or both. Because the functions of nerves III, IV, and VI and nerves IX and X overlap, assess these groups together.

CRANIAL NERVE I

To assess this nerve, which controls sense of smell, have the patient identify familiar odors with his eyes closed.

CRANIAL NERVE II

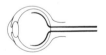

Before assessing the *optic nerve*, inspect the eyes for cataracts, inflammation, or corneal scarring. Then test visual acuity with a Snellen's chart or newspaper. Also test visual fields.

CRANIAL NERVES III, IV, VI

Cranial nerve III, the *oculomotor nerve*, controls pupillary constriction, upper eyelid elevation, and most eye movements.

Cranial nerve IV, the *trochlear nerve*, controls downward and inward eye movements.

Cranial nerve VI, the *abducens nerve*, controls lateral eye movements. To assess this group of nerves, first inspect the eyelids for ptosis. Then assess ocular movements and note any eye deviation. Test accommodation and direct and consensual light reflexes.

CRANIAL NERVE V

This nerve imparts sensation to the corneas, nasal and oral

Continued

Guide to Cranial Nerve Assessment
Continued

CRANIAL NERVE V
Continued

mucosa, and facial skin. It also controls the muscles of mastication. To assess its function, first have the patient close his eyes. Touch his jaws, cheeks, and forehead bilaterally with a cotton wisp and then with the point of a pin. Next, lightly touch the cornea with a cotton wisp. Have the patient clench his jaw. Palpate the temporal and masseter muscles bilaterally. Try to separate the patient's clenched jaw to test muscle strength. Finally, observe for asymmetry as the patient clenches and unclenches his jaw.

CRANIAL NERVE VII

This nerve controls all facial muscles. It's also responsible for taste perception on the anterior portion of the tongue. To assess its function, have the patient smile, show his teeth, and puff out his cheeks. Then observe for facial symmetry as the patient raises and lowers his eyebrows. Have the patient identify sugar, salt, vinegar, and a bitter substance placed on the anterior portion of the tongue.

CRANIAL NERVE VIII

The cochlear division of this nerve controls hearing; the vestibular division controls equilibrium, body position, and orientation to space. To screen for hearing loss, occlude one ear and whisper near the other. Ask the patient if he can hear you. To evaluate hearing more precisely, perform the Weber's, Rinne, or Schwabach tests. Have an audiologist perform caloric testing to assess the vestibular division.

CRANIAL NERVES IX, X

Cranial nerve IX, the *glossopharyngeal nerve*, controls swallowing and supplies sensation to the mucous membranes of the pharynx. It's also responsible for taste

Continued

Guide to Cranial Nerve Assessment
Continued

CRANIAL NERVES IX AND X
Continued

perception on the posterior third of the tongue and for salivation.

Cranial nerve X, the *vagus nerve*, controls swallowing, phonation, and movement of the uvula and soft palate. It also supplies sensation to the mucosa of the pharynx, soft palate, tonsils, and viscera of the thorax and abdomen. To assess the function of these nerves, first have the patient identify tastes at the back of the tongue. Then inspect the soft palate. Observe for symmetrical elevation when the patient says "ahh." Touch the mucous membrane of the soft palate with a swab to elicit the palatal reflex. Touch the posterior pharyngeal wall with a tongue depressor to elicit the gag reflex.

CRANIAL NERVE XI

This nerve controls the ster-

nocleidomastoid muscles and the upper portion of the trapezius muscles. To assess its function, palpate and inspect the sternocleidomastoid muscle as the patient pushes his chin against your hand. Palpate and inspect the trapezius muscle as the patient shrugs his shoulders against your resistance. Also have the patient stretch out his hands toward you.

CRANIAL NERVE XII

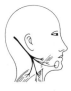

This nerve controls normal tongue movements involved in swallowing and speech. To assess its function, first observe the tongue for asymmetry, deviation to one side, loss of bulk, and fasciculations. Ask the patient to push his tongue against a tongue depressor. Then have him move his tongue rapidly in and out and from side to side.

Understanding Sympathetic and Parasympathetic Nervous Systems

The parasympathetic and sympathetic divisions of the autonomic nervous system play balancing roles in the regulation of the body's cardiac muscles, smooth muscles, and glands. To understand the effects of each division, review the following chart.

You should know that neurotransmitters must be present for any action to take place. The *parasympathetic* division, composed of cholinergic fibers, originates in the cranial area (CN III, VII, IX, and X) and the sacral area (S2 to S4) and uses acetylcholine as its neurotransmitter. The *sympathetic* division, composed of adrenergic fibers, originates in the thoracic area (T1 to T12) and the lumbar area (L1 to L3) and uses epinephrine and norepinephrine as its neurotransmitters.

ORGAN AFFECTED	PARASYMPA-THETIC EFFECTS	SYMPATHETIC EFFECTS
Pupil	• Contraction of sphincter muscle; pupil constricts	• Contraction of dilator muscle; pupil dilates
Ciliary muscle	• Contraction; accommodation for near vision	• Relaxation; accommodation for distant vision
Lacrimal gland	• Secretion	• Excessive secretion
Salivary glands	• Copious secretion of watery saliva	• Scanty, thick secretion of mucus-rich saliva
Respiratory system **Trachea/bronchial tree** **Blood vessels**	• Contraction of smooth muscle; decreased diameters and volumes • Little effect	• Relaxation of smooth muscle; increased diameters and volumes • Mildly constricted

Continued

PATIENT EVALUATION

Understanding Sympathetic and Parasympathetic Nervous Systems
Continued

ORGAN AFFECTED	PARASYMPA-THETIC EFFECTS	SYMPATHETIC EFFECTS
Heart		
Rate	• Decreased	• Increased
Stroke volume	• Decreased	• Increased
Cardiac output and blood pressure	• Decreased	• Increased
Coronary vessels	• Constriction	• Dilation
Peripheral blood vessels		
Skeletal muscle	• No innervation	• Dilation
Skin	• No innervation	• Constriction
Visceral organs (except heart and lungs)	• Dilation	• Constriction (may be insignificant)
Stomach		
Wall	• Increased motility	• Decreased motility
Sphincters	• Relaxed	• Contracted
Glands	• Increased secretion	• Decreased secretion
Intestines		
Wall	• Increased motility	• Decreased motility
Sphincters (pyloric, iliocecal, and internal anal)	• Inhibited	• Stimulated
Liver	• Promotes glycogenesis; increases bile secretion	• Promotes glycogenolysis; decreases bile secretion

Continued

Understanding Sympathetic and Parasympathetic Nervous Systems
Continued

ORGAN AFFECTED	PARASYMPA-THETIC EFFECTS	SYMPATHETIC EFFECTS
Pancreas (exocrine and endocrine)	• Increased secretion	• Decreased secretion
Spleen	• Little effect	• Contraction and emptying of stored blood into circulation
Adrenal medulla	• Little effect	• Norepinephrine/epi-nephrine secretion
Urinary bladder	• Stimulates wall; relaxes sphincter	• Inhibits wall; con-tracts sphincter
Uterus	• Little effect	• Inhibits motility of nonpregnant organ; stimulates pregnant organ
Penis	• Erection	• Ejaculation
Skeletal muscles	• No effect	• Increases glycoge-nolysis
Skin	• Little effect	• Constriction
Sweat glands	• No innervation	• Increases secretion
Kidneys	• No effect	• Decreased urinary output

Adapted from J. Robert McClintic, *Physiology of the Human Body* (2nd ed.; New York; John Wiley & Sons Publishers, 1978), with permission of the publisher.

Routine Skull Series

Right lateral and left lateral

The sagittal plane is parallel to the tabletop and the film. A support, such as the patient's clenched fist, or a folded towel, is placed under the chin. (Adequate film shows both halves of the mandible directly superimposed.)

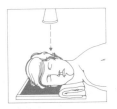

Posteroanterior (PA) Caldwell

The patient lies prone (his chin may be supported with his fist or a folded towel). The sagittal plane and the canthomeatal line are perpendicular to the tabletop and the film. The X-ray beam is angled 15° toward the feet.

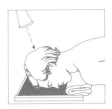

Anteroposterior (AP) Towne's

The patient lies supine, with his chin flexed toward the neck. The canthomeatal line is perpendicular to the tabletop and the film. The X-ray beam is angled 30° toward the feet.

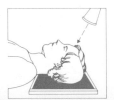

Axial (base)

The patient lies prone, with chin fully extended; his head rests in such a way that the line of the face is perpendicular and the canthomeatal line is parallel to the tabletop and the film.

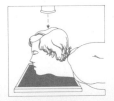

EEGs: Recording the Brain's Electrical Activity

In electroencephalography (EEG), electrodes attached to the patient's scalp, as shown, detect electrical impulses generated by the brain's nerve cells. Lead wires then transmit these impulses to an EEG machine, which translates them into waveforms. Among the basic waveforms are the alpha, beta, theta, and delta rhythms. Alpha waves occur at frequencies of 8 to 12 cycles/second in a regular rhythm and are most prominent in the occipital region of the brain. They're present only in the waking state when the patient's eyes are closed but he's mentally alert; usually, they disappear with visual activity or mental concentration. Beta waves (13 to 30 cycles/second)—generally associated with anxiety, depression, or sedative drugs—are seen most readily in the frontal and central regions of the brain. Theta waves (4 to 7 cycles/second) are most common in children and young adults and appear in the frontal and temporal regions. Delta waves (0.5 to 3.5 cycles/second) normally occur only in young children and during sleep.

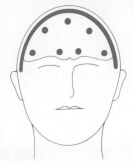

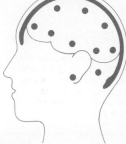

Beta waves

Theta waves

Alpha waves

Delta waves

Viewing the Brain's Interior

Advances in research and technology continue to refine and develop safer, more rewarding methods for studying the nervous system. Computerized tomography (CT), positron emission tomography (PET), and, more recently, magnetic resonance imaging (MRI) are major strides in noninvasive neurodiagnostic testing.

Computerized tomography

CT is a noninvasive test that provides clear, cross-sectional images of the head and spine, based on computer reconstruction of radiation levels absorbed by various tissues. The reconstructed image displays tissue density within a black-to-white spectrum. Black areas on the CT scan correspond to air density; white areas, to bone and blood density. Shades of gray correspond to cerebrospinal fluid and soft-tissue density. Valuable for diagnosing intracranial and spinal lesions, the CT scan also helps identify hydrocephalus, cerebral atrophy, and cerebral edema.

Positron emission tomography

Like CT scanning, PET provides cross-sectional images of the head but involves a different technique. This experimental test maps the brain's metabolic activity by recording gamma rays produced by the union of an injected biochemical—typically glucose—tagged with a radioisotope and negatively charged electrons in the brain. Abnormal isotope concentration identifies brain areas damaged by stroke or contusion or areas involved in seizure activity. Current research aims to understand the interaction of neurotransmitters in the brain. Locating dopamine and its receptor sites, for example, may provide an effective treatment or cure for Parkinson's disease.

Differentiating Between Invasive Tests

During diagnostic testing, the doctor will probably order several invasive tests. Which tests will the doctor order? That depends on your patient's condition, the doctor's preference, and your hospital's equipment.

Invasive neurologic testing can be frightening to both your patient and his family. So much depends on how well you prepare them before testing. For example, do you know how to explain a lumbar puncture to your patient? Your step-by-step details and emotional support will help him understand the procedure as well as what's expected of him. Or, in another case, your description of angiography and the importance of postprocedural bed rest may minimize complications.

Be completely prepared the next time you care for a patient scheduled for neurologic testing. Learn all you can about invasive testing procedures. Study the charts on these pages to find out how to properly prepare, monitor, and care for your patient before and after these test procedures.

LUMBAR PUNCTURE

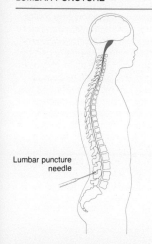

Lumbar puncture needle

• A percutaneous puncture entering the spinal column's subarachnoid space at the vertebral interspace L_3-L_4 or L_4-L_5. A lumbar puncture is performed for cerebrospinal fluid (CSF) pressure measurement; withdrawal of a CSF specimen for analysis; and the introduction of contrast media for diagnostic tests.

Indications

• To reduce intracranial pressure (ICP) after a spontaneous hemorrhage, by releasing CSF.

• To help diagnose diffuse or disseminated infections of the nervous system or meninges; subarachnoid hemorrhage; or demyelinating diseases.

• To introduce anesthetic, antibiotics, or other therapeutic drugs into the area.

Continued

Differentiating Between Invasive Tests
Continued

LUMBAR PUNCTURE
Continued

• To identify degree of subarachnoid blockage.

Special considerations
• Do not perform when increased ICP may be caused by an expanding lesion, such as a subdural hematoma after a head injury.
• Perform cautiously in patient with suspected spinal cord or brain tumor. Procedure may cause fatal cerebellar tonsillar herniation or compression of medulla.
• After the procedure, keep patient flat in bed for 4 to 6 hours. Encourage him to drink plenty of fluids.
• Observe puncture site for edema, hematoma, and CSF leakage.
• Perform a neurocheck, as ordered or indicated.

PNEUMOENCEPHALOGRAPHY

• Infusion of a gas such as air, nitrous oxide, or oxygen, through a lumbar or cisternal puncture. A series of X-rays taken during the infusion allows the doctor to visualize the ventricular system and meningeal spaces. In some hospitals, angiography and computer-

ized tomography have replaced this test, but it remains a valuable diagnostic tool for certain types of lesions.

Indications
• To identify lesions by determining ventricular size, shape, and position.

Special considerations
• Administer medications as needed for headache, nausea, vomiting, diaphoresis, and dizziness.
• Keep patient flat in bed for 24 to 48 hours. Every 2 hours, change your patient's position from side to side.
• Unless your patient complains of nausea, encourage him to drink plenty of fluids and eat foods high in sodium. Doing so replaces CSF and promotes reabsorption of the infused air.
• Notify the doctor if you note increased ICP, seizures, shock, prolonged or intractable headache, nausea, vomiting, chills, or fever.

MYELOGRAPHY

• Infusion of dye or gas into spinal column's subarachnoid space through a lumbar puncture. A series of X-rays taken during the infusion allows the doctor to visualize the spinal column.

Indications
• To identify space-occupying le-
Continued

Differentiating Between Invasive Tests
Continued

MYELOGRAPHY
Continued

sions of the spinal cord.
• To help diagnose a herniated nucleus pulposus.

Special considerations
• Administer medications, as ordered, for headache, nausea, vomiting, diaphoresis, and dizziness.
• Keep patient in bed for 24 to 48 hours, as ordered. Elevate the head of his bed, as ordered.
• Perform a neurocheck, as ordered.
• Unless your patient feels nauseated, encourage him to drink plenty of fluids and eat foods high in sodium.
• Notify the doctor if you note increased ICP, seizures, shock, prolonged or intractable headache, nausea, vomiting, chills, or fever.

CISTERNAL PUNCTURE

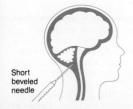

Short beveled needle

• A puncture entering the subarachnoid space between the cerebellum and the medulla (cisterna magna) located between the first cervical lamina and the ridge of the foramen magnum. Insertion of a short, beveled needle allows for CSF pressure measurements; CSF withdrawal for analysis; and introduction of contrast media for diagnostic tests.

Indications
• Performed when a lumbar puncture's contraindicated or a subarachnoid block exists.
• To reduce ICP.
• To help diagnose: diffuse or disseminated infections of the nervous system or meninges; a subarachnoid hemorrhage; or a demyelinating disease.

Special considerations
• Assess patient frequently for signs and symptoms of cerebellar tonsillar medullary herniation, such as nuchal rigidity, motor paralysis, jackknife spasticity, hyperactive deep tendon reflexes in involved limb, medullary collapse, or circulatory collapse.

Continued

Differentiating Between Invasive Tests
Continued

VENTRICULOGRAPHY

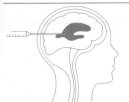

• Infusion of air or dye into the lateral ventricle through a puncture in the skull. A series of X-rays taken during the infusion allows the doctor to visualize the ventricular and meningeal vascular systems. Performed when a lumbar or cisternal puncture is contraindicated to relieve elevated ICP.

Indications
• To ensure ventricular system patency.
• To establish ventricular drainage.
• To identify and localize lesions and tumors.
• To identify cerebral anomalies.

Special considerations
• Prepare patient for surgery, as ordered. In many cases, a craniotomy follows this procedure.
• If ventricular tube must remain in place after the procedure, maintain a sterile closed system.
• Notify the doctor if you note hemorrhage, respiratory distress, increased ICP, seizures, hypovolemic shock, prolonged headache, nausea, vomiting, chills, or fever.
• Be sure to have a lumbar puncture tray at the patient's bedside in case a lumbar puncture is indicated to relieve sudden increased CSF pressure.
• Administer medications as ordered, for headache, nausea, vomiting, diaphoresis, and dizziness.
• Keep patient flat in bed for 24 to 48 hours. Elevate patient's head 15 to 20 degrees. Every 2 hours, change your patient's position from side to side.
• Encourage your patient to drink plenty of fluids, and eat foods high in sodium, if he can.

CEREBRAL ANGIOGRAPHY

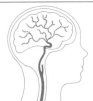

• Infusion of dye through a catheter directly or indirectly into the arterial system. A series of X-rays

Continued

Differentiating Between Invasive Tests
Continued

CEREBRAL ANGIOGRAPHY
Continued

taken during the infusion allows the doctor to visualize the cerebral vasculature.

Indications

• To identify cerebral circulatory anomalies, such as a subdural hematoma, epidural hematoma, massive intracranial lesion, cerebral edema, carotid-cavernous sinus fistula, or aneurysm.

Special considerations

• Keep patient in bed for 24 to 48 hours, as ordered.

• Monitor vital signs and perform a neurocheck, as ordered.

• Notify the doctor if you note puncture site hemorrhage, hematoma, signs of increased ICP, seizures, nausea, vomiting, chills, or fever.

• Apply ice packs to puncture site, as ordered.

• Check patient's circulation, as well as his ability to move.

• Encourage patient to drink plenty of fluids, unless he feels nauseated.

• Administer medications, as ordered, for headache, nausea, vomiting, diaphoresis, and dizziness.

BRAIN SCAN

• Infusion of a radioactive isotope I.V. A scintillation scanner measures the isotope's radiation emission and transmits a brain image onto a videoscreen. The isotope will accumulate in abnormal or damaged brain tissue.

Indications

• To identify intracranial diseases, such as gliomas and astrocytomas.

• To detect any remaining or spreading malignant tumors, following radiotherapy, chemotherapy, or a craniotomy.

Special considerations

• Assure your patient that the procedure is hazard-free. The isotope contains less radioactivity than X-rays.

• Tell the patient that repeat scans are usually necessary. Inform him that follow-up scans help the doctor monitor progress.

ELECTROMYOGRAPHY

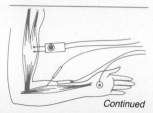

Continued

Differentiating Between Invasive Tests
Continued

ELECTROMYOGRAPHY
Continued

• Insertion of a surface needle or electrode into a skeletal muscle. An oscilloscope records subsequent electrical activity for audio and visual analysis.
Indications
• To identify and localize lower motor neuron diseases, such as muscular dystrophy.
• To assess the status of peripheral nerve reinnervation.
Special considerations
• Advise patient to expect some muscle tenderness after the test.
• Administer ice packs, as necessary.

Tensilon Test

In this test, after I.V. administration of Tensilon (edophonium chloride), an examiner observes and records the patient's motor response. The examiner asks the patient to make repetitive muscular movements such as opening and closing his eyes and crossing and uncrossing his legs. Tensilon, a rapid, short-acting anticholinesterase, improves muscle strength by increasing muscular response to nerve impulses.
Indications
• To help diagnose myasthenia gravis.
• To help differentiate between myasthenic and cholinergic crises.
• To monitor oral anticholinesterase therapy.
Special considerations
• Realize this test is often hard to interpret because Tensilon may improve function in one muscle group while increasing weakness in another muscle group. Therefore, to ensure accurate results, this test may be performed several times.
• Don't tell the patient the exact response that will be observed, since this information may interfere with the test's objectivity.
• Tell the patient that Tensilon may produce some unpleasant side effects—such as excessive sweating and salivation, abdominal cramping and tearing—but that these effects disappear quickly.
• Observe the patient closely for side effects.
• If the patient is receiving anticholinesterase therapy, note this and the amount and time of the last dose on the requisition slip.
• Make sure patients with respiratory disorders, such as asthma, receive atropine during the test to minimize Tensilon side effects.

Preparing for Cerebral Angiography

Is your patient scheduled for cerebral angiography? If so, begin your preprocedural preparation as soon as possible. To do so, follow these steps:

• Explain the procedure to your patient and answer any questions. Reassure him that the puncture area will be locally anesthetized so he should feel only slight discomfort during the procedure.

• Instruct the patient to fast for 8 to 10 hours before the test. Tell him who will perform the procedure and where.

• Make sure your patient's signed a consent form.

• Withhold foods and fluids for 6 hours prior to the procedure. Tell your patient these precautions reduce the risk of nausea or vomiting during the procedure.

• Check your patient's vital signs and perform a neurocheck routinely, or as ordered, to establish a data baseline.

• Ask the patient if he has any allergies, especially to shellfish or iodine. If he does, notify the doctor. Why? Because the dye infused during this test has an iodine base and a patient with these allergies may suffer anaphylaxis.

• Notify the doctor of any hypersensitivities; he may order prophylactic medications or he may choose not to perform the test.

• Explain to the patient that he'll probably feel a transient burning sensation as the contrast media is injected, that he may feel flushed and warm, and that he may experience a transient headache or salty taste after injection of the dye.

• Be sure a crash cart's handy. In rare cases, the dye used during the procedure may produce respiratory distress and anaphylactic shock.

• If the puncture site is located on the patient's groin or other hairy area, shave the site, according to your hospital's policy. Be sure to explain to the patient why shaving's necessary.

• Document all preprocedural teaching and preparations in your nurses' notes.

What Can Cerebrospinal Fluid (CSF) Tell You?

Consider this: Several hours ago, the doctor performed a lumbar puncture on your patient. Now you're attaching the completed lab slip to your patient's chart. Wondering what these diagnostic test results mean?

	INTRACRANIAL ABSCESS	INTRACRANIAL TUMOR
Pressure Normal range is from 60 to 180 mm water	• Elevated	• Elevated
Appearance Normally clear	• Clear, but may be discolored if abscess ruptures	• Clear
Cellular makeup Normal is 0 to 5 lymphocytes	• Amount varies from normal to increased	• Increased
Protein Normal is 15 to 45 mg per 100 ml	• Results vary from normal to increased	• Increased
Glucose Normal is 60% to 80% of true blood sugar; 40 to 80 mg per 100 ml	• Results vary from normal to decreased	• Normal

Although interpreting results from cerebrospinal fluid (CSF) samples is the doctor's responsibility, you can learn to identify the characteristics of some common disorders. Use the chart below as a guide.

CEREBRAL INFARCT	SUBARACHNOID HEMORRHAGE	ACUTE BACTERIAL MENINGITIS
• Elevated	• Readings vary from normal to extreme elevation	• Readings vary from moderate to extreme elevation
• Usually clear	• Pink to red	• Clear to purulent
• Slightly increased	• Increase in red and white blood cells	• Increase in white blood cells, usually between 10,000 to 50,000
• Slightly increased	• Increased	• Increased
• Normal	• Results vary from normal to marked decrease	• Decreased

PATIENT EVALUATION

Nursing Role in Diagnostic Tests

What's your role when it comes to diagnostic tests? Although you probably won't be with the patient when he undergoes each test, you will need to prepare him for it and care for him afterwards. Here are the general guidelines:

• Teach your patient all he needs to know about the test. Tell him what sensations and reactions he can expect to get during the test. Stress the importance of following instructions and staying in the correct position. Encourage questions so you can clear up any misconceptions.

• Prepare your patient physically. This preparation varies from test to test. Noninvasive tests, such as skull and spinal X-rays, usually require no physical preparation. However, an invasive test may require 1) written permit signed by patient or appropriate person; 2) baseline vital signs and neurologic assessment; 3) complete restriction of oral intake for specified time; 4) medications, as ordered; 5) removal of prostheses, as well as such items as hairpins and jewelry.

• Understand the risks involved with each test. Watch for signs of complications, but prevent them when possible.

• Give your patient the care he needs after his test. Observe closely for changes in vital signs and neurologic status.

Diagnostic Testing in Degenerative Disease

ALZHEIMER'S DISEASE

X-rays
Normal
Myelography
Normal
Cerebrospinal fluid
Normal
CT scan
Symmetrically enlarged ventricles with widening of cortical sulci

Blood and urine studies
Normal
Brain biopsy
Neurofibrillary tangles and plaques with positive fuchsin staining
EEG
Diffuse slowing in advanced disease
Other studies
Frontal and temporal lobe atrophy on pneumoencephalogram

Continued

Diagnostic Testing in Degenerative Disease
Continued

AMYTROPHIC LATERAL SCLEROSIS (ALS)

X-rays
Normal
Myelography
Normal
Cerebrospinal fluid
Normal
CT scan
Normal
Electromyography
Fibrillation potentials and a decreased number of motor units; nerve conduction normal
Blood studies
Creatine phosphokinase (CPK) normal or slightly increased
Urine studies
Increased creatine
Decreased creatinine
Muscle biopsy
Small, angulated atrophic fibers in groups
Other studies
Decreased strength in serial muscle testing, decreased pulmonary function in pulmonary function tests, decreased swallowing ability on fluoroscopy.

HUNTINGTON'S CHOREA

X-rays
Normal
Cerebrospinal fluid
Decreased gamma-aminobutyric acid
CT scan
Ventricular dilation
Blood and urine studies
Normal
EEG
Loss and slowing of alpha activity

PARKINSON'S DISEASE

X-rays
Normal
Cerebrospinal fluid
Normal or decreased dopamine and its metabolites
CT scan
Ventricular dilation possible with diffuse cortical atrophy
Electromyography
Normal
Blood and urine studies
Normal
EEG
Diffuse, nonspecific slowing of theta waves
Other studies
Tremor studies, decreased performance in serial measurements of functional activity

MULTIPLE SCLEROSIS (MS)

X-rays
Normal

Continued

Diagnostic Testing in Degenerative Disease
Continued

MULTIPLE SCLEROSIS (MS)
Continued

Myelography
Enlarged spinal cord possible
Cerebrospinal fluid
Myelin, basic protein fractions, oligoclonal bands, increased IgG in 66% of cases, slight increase in white cells
CT scan
Increased tissue density of white matter
Visual-evoked potentials
Abnormal in about 94% of cases
Electromyography
Abnormal in advanced stages
Blood and urine studies
Normal
EEG
Possible nonspecific abnormalities
Other studies
Positive electronystagmography, decreased performance in serial measurements of functional activity

TAY-SACHS DISEASE

X-rays
Normal
Myelography
Normal
Cerebrospinal fluid
Increased SGOT, SGPT, LDH
CT scan
Ventricular atrophy with widening of sulci
Blood studies
Increased SGOT, SGPT, LDH, CPK; decreased hexosaminidase A; large azurophilic granules in lymphocyte smears of peripheral blood
Urine studies
Normal
Brain biopsy
Neurons distended with lipids, nucleus at cell periphery, and loss of Nissl bodies
EEG
Abnormal when vision loss occurs
Other studies
Rectal biopsy with abnormal lipid accumulation in neurons of Auerbach's and Meissner's plexus; decreased hexosaminidase A in skin biopsy and tissue cultures of fibroblasts

WERDNIG-HOFFMAN

X-rays
Normal
Myelography
Normal
Cerebrospinal fluid
Normal
Electromyography
Abnormal
Blood studies
Increased SGOT, SGPT, LDH, and CPK
Urine studies
Myoglobinuria, creatine, creatinine
Muscle biopsy
Abnormal

Disorders in Transmission of Nerve Impulses

SYRINGOMYELIA

Chief complaint
• *Headache/pain*: painful shoulder
• *Motor disturbances*: weakness; hyporeflexia, hyperreflexia, or areflexia; wasting of muscles at level of spinal cord involvement (usually hands and arms); spasticity of lower levels; nystagmus; atrophy and fibrillation of the tongue
• *Sensory deviations*: anesthesia in hands or face
History
• Onset usually between ages 30 and 50
• Symptoms include spontaneous fractures, painless injuries, ulcers from anesthesia; progress irregular (may be in remission for long period)
Physical examination
• Horner's syndrome, nystagmus, knee or shoulder joint deformities, clonus, spasticity, hyperreflexia
• Loss of deep tendon reflex, gradual loss of pain and temperature sense

MYASTHENIA GRAVIS

Chief complaint
• *Motor disturbances*: progressive muscle weakness during activity; respiratory muscles affected during crisis; dysarthria; dysphagia
• *Sensory deviations*: double vision, weak eye muscles

History
• Onset usually between ages 20 and 40
• Most common in females
• Remissions and exacerbations common
• Symptoms worsen with emotional stress, prolonged exposure to sunlight or cold
Physical examination
• Deep tendon reflexes present
• Double vision, weak eye closure; ptosis; expressionless face; nasal vocal tones; nasal regurgitation of fluids; weak chewing muscles; weak respiratory muscles; weak neck muscles, can't support head; proximal limb weakness (may be asymmetrical)

POLYNEURITIS

Chief complaint
• *Motor disturbances*: leg weakness or paralysis progressing to arms and trunk; weakness most severe in distal extremities and in extensors; footdrop; ataxia; absent leg reflexes; impairment of bowel and bladder function and sphincter control
• *Sensory deviations*: paresthesias in hands or feet; anesthesia or hyperesthesia in distal parts of arms and legs; impaired vibratory and kinesthetic sensibilities; nerves sensitive to pressure

Continued

Disorders in Transmission of Nerve Impulses
Continued

POLYNEURITIS
Continued

History
● Precipitating factors include alcohol abuse, inadequate diet and malnutrition, pregnancy, gastrointestinal disorders, vitamin B deficiency, weight loss
● Common in diabetics over age 50
Physical examination
● Dry, scaly skin on back of wrists and hands, hyperpigmentation of skin, plantar responses absent, abdominal skin reflexes decreased or absent, increased pulse rate possible; reduced or absent patellar and Achilles tendon reflex
● Feet tender in diabetics

WERNICKE'S ENCEPHALOPATHY

Chief complaint
● *Motor disturbances*: ophthalmoplegia, ataxia, nystagmus, tremors
● *Seizures*: may occur
● *Sensory deviations*: paresthesias of hands and feet
● *Altered level of consciousness*: drowsiness; impaired recent memory; unaffected remote, past memory; confabulation; time disorientation; apathy; mild lethargy; occasional frank delirium

History
● Predisposing factors include inadequate diet, low thiamine intake, and alcohol addiction.
● Pernicious vomiting possible during pregnancy
Physical examination
● Mental disturbance, retrograde or anterograde amnesia, paralysis of eye movements, ataxia, diplopia, nystagmus, broad-based stance

LANDRY'S OR GUILLAIN-BARRÉ SYNDROME (acute idiopathic polyneuritis)

Chief complaint
● *Motor disturbances*: muscle weakness in legs, extending to arms and face in 24 to 72 hours and progressing to total paralysis and respiratory failure; flaccid quadriplegia possible; cranial nerve paralysis; ocular paralysis in about 25% of cases
● *Sensory deviations*: paresthesias vanishing before muscle weakness occurs
History
● Onset at any age
● Predisposing factors include recent viral or bacterial infection, surgery, influenza vaccination, Hodgkin's disease, lupus erythematosus, gastroenteritis
● Rapid onset of muscular symptoms

Continued

NEUROLOGIC DISORDERS

Disorders in Transmission of Nerve Impulses
Continued

LANDRY'S OR GUILLAIN-
BARRÉ SYNDROME
Continued

Physical examination
• Retinal hemorrhage, sinus tachycardia or bradycardia, choked disk, hypertension, signs of increased intracranial pressure, elevated cerebrospinal fluid pressure, cranial nerve paralysis (VII), symmetrical loss of tendon reflexes, ascending peripheral nerve paralysis or weakness, impaired proprioception, loss of bowel and bladder control, muscle tenderness to pressure

MULTIPLE SCLEROSIS (disseminated sclerosis)

Chief complaint
• *Motor disturbances:* slurred speech, intention tremor, nystagmus (Charcot's triad), spastic paralysis, poor coordination, loss of proprioception, ataxia, transient muscle weakness, incontinence or retention
• *Sensory deviations:* numbness and tingling, vision impairment
• *Altered level of consciousness:* euphoria, emotionally unstable
History
• Most common in young white adults
• Higher incidence in northern climate

• Genetic tendencies
• Initial attack and subsequent relapse may follow acute infections, trauma, vaccination, serum injections, pregnancy, stress.
Physical examination
• Pale optic disk on temporal side, increased deep tendon reflexes, joint contractures and deformities, scanning speech, cranial nerve involvement (vertigo, trigeminal neuralgia), decreased or diminished abdominal reflexes, unsteady gait

GRAND MAL SEIZURE (major motor, generalized, tonic clonic)

Chief conplaint
• *Headache:* present on awakening, possibly accompanied by nausea
• *Motor disturbances:* generalized tonic and clonic movements; residual hemiparesis or monoparesis possible
• *Seizures:* generalized
• *Sensory deviations:* weakness, dizziness, numbness, peculiar sensation
• *Altered level of consciousness:* loss of consciousness; mental confusion after awakening, lasting several hours or days
History
• Onset early in life with idiopathic disorder; can occur at any
Continued

NEUROLOGIC DISORDERS

Disorders in Transmission of Nerve Impulses
Continued

GRAND MAL SEIZURE
Continued

age with secondary disorders, but those associated with fever commonly occur in children
• Predisposing factors include, with idiopathic seizure disorders (epilepsy), familial history of seizures, genetic involvement; with secondary seizure disorders, cerebral palsy, birth injury, infectious diseases, meningitis, encephalitis, cerebral trauma, metabolic disturbances, cerebral edema, carbon monoxide poisoning, insulin shock, anoxia, brain tumor, drug overdose, child abuse, noncompliance with medication regimen
Physical examination
• Shrill cry, pupillary change, loss of consciousness, tonic and clonic movements, tongue-biting, abnormal respiratory pattern (absent during tonic phase), urinary or fecal incontinence, upward deviation of eyes, excessive salivation

JACKSONIAN SEIZURE (partial motor and partial sensory)

Chief complaint
• *Motor disturbances*: focal seizures, lesions of motor cortex or strip (jacksonian motor seizure)
• *Seizures*: partial, with no loss of consciousness
• *Sensory deviations*: numbness, tingling of one arm or leg or one half of body, auditory alterations (such as ringing noises), lesions of the sensory strip (jacksonian sensory seizure)
History
• Predisposing factors include birth injury, trauma, infection, and vascular lesions.
Physical examination
• Clonic twitching begins in one part of body, usually one side of the face or the fingers of one hand, and often progresses from face to hand, to arm, to trunk, to legs on the same side of the body (jacksonian march); if twitching begins in the foot, it may progress reversely through the body; rhythmic clonic movements may affect one area (face, arm, leg) without marching.
• Speech loss possible
• Sensory deviations may also progress or march through the body.
• May progress to a secondary generalized seizure (grand mal)

PSYCHOMOTOR SEIZURE (focal)

Chief complaint
• *Motor disturbances*: speech disturbance; destructive, aggressive behavior
• *Seizures*: temporal lobe dysfunction (behavior disturbance)
• *Sensory deviations*: olfactory
Continued

Disorders in Transmission of Nerve Impulses
Continued

PSYCHOMOTOR SEIZURE
Continued

hallucinations and other sensory manifestations depending on location of focus; feeling of déjà vu and déjà pensé
● *Altered level of consciousness:* slower thought processes; altered consciousness; partial amnesia
History
● Secondary to birth injury or congenital abnormalities in infants, lesions or trauma in children and adults, arteriosclerosis in adults
Physical examination
● Aura may occur in the form of a hallucination or perceptual illusion
● May begin with aura
● Characterized by automatisms (patterned behavior): lip-smacking, head-turning, dressing, undressing
● Extreme psychotic behavior possible

AMYOTROPHIC LATERAL SCLEROSIS (Lou Gehrig's disease)

Chief complaint
● *Headache/pain:* pain in arms and legs
● *Motor disturbances:* muscle atrophy and weakness, especially in forearms and hands; fasciculations; impaired speech; difficulty chewing, swallowing, and breathing; choking; excessive drooling; urinary frequency, urgency, and difficulty initiating a stream; in advanced disease flaccid quadriplegia, dysphagia, and muscle weakness
● *Sensory deviations:* paresthesias
● *Altered level of consciousness:* depression; crying spells and inappropriate laughter caused by bulbar palsy
History
● Onset usually between ages 40 and 70
● Most common in white males
● Precipitating factors include nutritional deficiency, vitamin E deficiency (damaging cell membranes), autoimmune disorder, interference with nucleic acid production, acute viral infections, and physical exhaustion.
● Usually fatal in 2 to 3 years, usually a result of aspiration pneumonia or respiratory failure.
● In 10% of patients, ALS is inherited as an autosomal dominant trait.
Physical examination
● Deep tendon reflexes absent; muscle twitches

When Your Patient Goes into Myasthenia Gravis Crisis

Are you familiar with the nursing interventions for a patient in myasthenia gravis crisis? Can you differentiate the myasthenic type from the cholinergic? This chart shows you the causes and signs and symptoms of each type of myasthenia gravis crisis, along with appropriate nursing interventions.

NEUROLOGIC DISORDERS

MYASTHENIC CRISIS

Mechanisms
• Respiratory muscles weaken, causing respiratory failure.

Signs and symptoms
• Acute respiratory distress with irritability, anxiety, extreme restlessness, decreased urine output, increased pulse, diminished cough and swallow reflexes, difficulty speaking, double vision, drooping eyelids, increased salivation
• Positive response to Tensilon test—muscle strength improves

Nursing considerations
• Be prepared to ventilate and suction your patient.
• Be prepared to assist with a tracheotomy or with insertion of an endotracheal tube.
• Monitor his vital signs.
• Be prepared to administer anticholinesterase agents, such as neostigmine or pyridostigmine, to improve neuromuscular transmission.

CHOLINERGIC CRISIS

Mechanisms
• Too much anticholinesterase medication causes respiratory failure.

Causes
• Overmedication with cholinergic drugs

Signs and symptoms
• Extreme weakness with difficulty speaking; diminished cough and swallow reflexes with increased salivation; acute respiratory distress; micosis; nausea; vomiting; diarrhea; abdominal cramps; fine muscle tremors of eyelids, face, neck, or legs; bradycardia; pallor; sweating
• Negative response to Tensilon test—signs and symptoms worsen

Nursing considerations
• Be prepared to ventilate and suction your patient.
• Be prepared to assist with a tracheotomy or with insertion of an endotracheal tube.
• Monitor his vital signs.
• Discontinue use of anticholinesterase drugs during the crisis until his condition improves.
• Be prepared to administer I.V. injection of 1 mg atropine to counteract the muscarinic effects of the severe cholinergic reaction.

What Happens in Myasthenia Gravis

As you probably know, myasthenia gravis is a chronic disease that produces recurrent, progressive attacks of muscle weakness and abnormal fatigability. Exercise worsens these signs and symptoms.

A disturbance in nerve impulse transmission at the neuromuscular junction affects muscle contraction. Although the exact mechanism's unknown, researchers believe it involves insufficient acetylcholine synthesis, re-

lease, or binding at the neuromuscular junction. A widely accepted theory postulates the cause of myasthenia gravis to be an autoimmune disorder in which antibodies destroy many postsynaptic receptor sites in muscle fiber membranes. The synapse widens, and the number of clefts decreases. Affected muscles are unable to contract normally. (See illustration.)

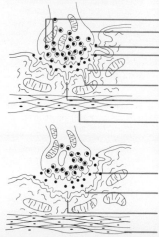

NORMAL NEUROMUSCULAR JUNCTION
Vesicles
Nerve terminal
Acetylcholine
Synapse
Normal acetylcholine receptor
Subneural cleft
Muscle-fiber membrane with acetylcholine receptor
Muscle fibers

NEUROMUSCULAR JUNCTION AFFECTED BY MYASTHENIA GRAVIS
Widened synapse
Destroyed acetylcholine receptors
Destroyed subneural clefts
Damaged muscle fibers

Seizure Onset and Cause

AGE AT ONSET	USUAL CAUSE
0 to 2	Congenital defect, anoxia at birth, meningitis, hypocalcemia, hypoglycemia, vitamin B_6 deficiency, phenylketonuria
2 to 10	Anoxia or injury at birth, meningitis, infections, thrombosis of cerebral vessels, idiopathic epilepsy
10 to 18	Idiopathic epilepsy, trauma, meningitis, congenital defects
18 to 35	Idiopathic epilepsy, trauma, tumor, meningitis, withdrawal from alcohol or sedative-hypnotic drugs
35 to 60	Trauma, tumor, vascular disease, meningitis, alcohol or drug withdrawal
Over 60	Vascular disease, tumor, degenerative disease, meningitis

Phases of Seizure Activity

Prodromal. Mood or behavior change that may precede seizure by several hours or days.

Aura. Unusual sound, sight, taste, or smell, warning of impending seizure. Epileptic cry may occur.

Ictal. Seizure activity.

Postictal. After-seizure behavioral changes, lethargy, confusion.

Taking Seizure Precautions

Whenever you care for a patient with a head injury, you can minimize seizure risk by taking the following precautions.

• Administer anticonvulsant medications on time. Do not omit or increase medication.
• Be sure to use a rectal thermometer, not an oral one, on the seizure-prone patient.
• Pad side rails and headboard to protect him from injury.
• Keep the padded, long side rails in place if he has frequent or generalized seizures, or if he has severe muscle contractions.
• When a patient has an oral endotracheal tube in place, insert an airway to prevent the patient from occluding or biting the endotracheal tube during seizure activity, and to allow for suctioning.
• Keep suction equipment handy in case the patient's airway becomes clogged with oral secretions.
• Monitor the patient's cardiovascular and respiratory status closely to detect hypoxia, which may lead to increased seizure activity.
• Provide emotional support to the patient and family.
• Accompany the seizure-prone patient when he takes a walk.

Nursing Care During a Seizure

When your patient has a seizure, take these actions:
• Stay with him and call for assistance.
• Lay the patient flat on the bed or floor. Then, try to turn him on his side.
• Loosen tight clothing; for example, his collar and belt.
• Move objects out of the way to protect his head and limbs from injury.
• Guide his movements, if possible, but don't restrain him.
• Don't force open clenched teeth.

After your patient's seizure, take these actions:
• Place him in bed, if he isn't already.
• Ensure a patent airway by turning him on his side to permit oral drainage. Check his level of consciousness. If it's depressed, insert an oral airway. Suction, as needed.
• Notify the doctor immediately.
• Check the patient for injury.
• Reorient the patient as necessary.
• Document everything in your nurses' notes.

Differentiating Seizure Types

DISORDER/AREAS INVOLVED (FOCUS)	CHANGE IN CONSCIOUSNESS
I. Partial seizures (simple)	
A. Focal motor Motor strip on precentral gyrus in frontal lobe	Unilateral: No change in consciousness. Bilateral: Loss of consciousness
B. Jacksonian Motor strip on precentral gyrus in frontal lobe	Unilateral: No change in consciousness. Bilateral: Loss of consciousness
C. Adversive Frontal lobe anterior to motor strip	No loss
D. Epilepsia partialis continua Varied	No loss
E. Focal sensory Postcentral gyrus in parietal or occipital lobe	No loss
II. Partial seizures (complex)	
A. Psychomotor Temporal lobe	No loss of consciousness; confusion and amnesia

EEG FINDINGS	IMPAIRED CAPACITIES
Focal waves, slow waves, or spikes	Convulsive movements and temporary disturbance in motor capacity in body part controlled by that brain region
Focal waves, slow waves, or spikes	Disturbance in motor capacity. Seizure activity marches along limb or side of body in orderly progression
Focal waves, slow waves, or spikes	Disturbance in behavior and motor capacity. Head and eyes turn away from focal region; may develop into generalized seizure
Focal waves, slow waves, or spikes	Form of focal status epilepticus involving a muscle group. May last minutes to weeks with postictal weakness
Spikes and slow waves over epileptogenic focus in occipital or parietal areas	Subjective sensory experience; may be visual, auditory, olfactory, or somatosensory. Possible "marching" progression
Temporal spikes or slow waves	Hallucinations, dyscognitive states (déjà vu), automatism, and loss of awareness

NEUROLOGIC DISORDERS

Continued

Differentiating Seizure Types
Continued

DISORDER/AREAS INVOLVED (FOCUS)	CHANGE IN CONSCIOUSNESS
III. Generalized seizures	
A. Generalized tonic-clonic (grand mal) Generalized	Loss of consciousness with postictal sleeping
B. Absence (petit mal) Generalized	Transient losses of consciousness; no postictal state
C. Infantile spasms (salaam, head drop) Generalized	None; no postictal state
D. Myoclonic Generalized	Possible momentary loss of consciousness followed by confusion
E. Akinetic (drop attacks) Generalized, with brain stem involvement	None; no postictal state
IV. Miscellaneous	
A. Mixed Frontal, temporal, or occipital focus with generalized spread	Consistent with type of seizure

NEUROLOGIC DISORDERS

EEG FINDINGS	IMPAIRED CAPACITIES
Rapidly repeating spikes in tonic phase; spikes of slow waves in clonic phase	Major tonic muscular contraction followed by longer phase of clonic (jerking) contractions. Possible bowel and bladder control loss, weakness, injury, or learning disorders
Spikes and waves, three/second	Interference with conscious response to environment when uncontrolled; possible learning disorders
Multiple spikes and slow waves of large amplitude (hypsarrhythmia)	Jackknife, flexor spasms of extremities and head. Severe mental and developmental deficiencies
Findings similar to those for infantile spasms	Uncontrollable jerking movements of extremities or entire body
Normal to slow background with polyspike or multiple spike waves	Sudden postural tone loss. Possible intellectual, perceptual, and motor impairments
Spike, polyspike, or spike-wave patterns with progression of focus to a generalized pattern	Interferences with behavior, learning, or motor functions

NEUROLOGIC DISORDERS

EEG Tracings during Different Types of Seizures

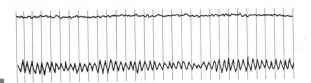

Normal (*Top: Right temporal; Bottom: Parietal-occipital*)

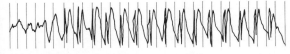

Petit mal epilepsy (*Spikes and waves, 3/second*)

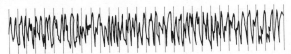

Grand mal epilepsy (*Multiple high-voltage spiked waves*)

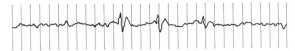

Right temporal lobe epilepsy (*Focal spiked waves*)

Disorders that Alter Protective Structures

MENINGITIS

Chief complaint
• *Headache*: present, with nausea and vomiting
• *Motor disturbances*: exaggerated, symmetrical deep tendon reflexes
• *Seizures*: may occur; generalized
• *Sensory deviations*: visual disturbances, such as photophobia
• *Altered level of consciousness*: irritability, confusion, stupor, or coma

History
• Predisposing factors include otitis media, mastoiditis, ruptured brain abscess, sinus infection, hepatitis, tonsillitis, herpes zoster or herpes simplex, bone or skin infection, heart valve or lung infection, skull fracture, recent surgery to head or face, recent viral or bacterial infection, general malaise.

Physical examination
• High- or low-grade fever, rash, sinus arrhythmias, photophobia, nuchal rigidity, opisthotonos, back pain, shock, signs of increased intracranial pressure, positive Brudzinski's and Kernig's signs

BRAIN ABSCESS

Chief complaint
• *Headache*: present, with nausea and vomiting
• *Motor disturbances*: hemiplegia, speech disturbances, cranial nerve palsies
• *Seizures*: focal or generalized
• *Sensory deviations*: visual field defect (hemianopia), depending on position of abscess
• *Altered level of consciousness*: behavioral changes or loss of consciousness

History
• Predisposing factors include mastoid and nasal sinus disease; bacterial endocarditis; pulmonary, skin, and abdominal infections; head trauma.

Physical examination
• Normal or decreased temperature, papilledema, signs of increased intracranial pressure
• Signs similar to those of meningitis, such as nuchal rigidity, positive Brudzinski's and Kernig's signs

ENCEPHALITIS

Chief complaint
• *Headache*: present
• *Motor disturbances*: residual Parkinsonian paralysis with acute attack; paralysis; ataxia
• *Seizures*: may occur during acute attack; residual seizures in about 60% of cases
• *Altered level of consciousness*: lethargy or restlessness progress-
Continued

Disorders that Alter Protective Structures
Continued

NEUROLOGIC DISORDERS

ENCEPHALITIS
Continued

ing to stupor and coma; may remain comatose several days, weeks, or longer after acute phase subsides; personality changes; mental deterioration in about 60% of cases

History
• Predisposing factors include mosquito bite, measles, chicken pox, mumps, herpes virus, polio vaccine or virus, syphilis (10 to 25 years after infection).

Physical examination
• Fever, nuchal rigidity, back pain, abnormal EEG, signs of increased intracranial pressure
• With history of syphilis, tremors, dysarthria, generalized convulsions, increased deep tendon reflexes, bilateral Babinski's sign; with history of herpes simplex, progressive confusion, recent memory loss, temporal lobe seizures, increased antibody levels to herpes simplex virus; with history of measles virus, memory impairment, seizures, myoclonic jerks, ataxia

HEAD INJURY

Chief complaint
• *Headache:* varies in intensity and duration; generalized, with nausea and vomiting
• *Motor disturbances:* specific to area of injury; dysphagia; dysarthria; paralysis; ataxia
• *Sensory deviation:* vertigo, tinnitus worsened by change in posture
• *Altered level of consciousness:* unconsciousness varies in depth and duration, depending on severity and area of injury (the more severe the injury, the greater the depth and duration of unconsciousness); confusion after regaining consciousness (the greater the duration of unconsciousness, the greater the incidence of permanent brain damage)

History
• Some type of fall or accident, such as a vehicular or industrial accident; blow to the head

Physical examination
• Signs of increased intracranial pressure, retrograde and post-traumatic amnesia, hyperthermia, shock, scalp bleeding, evidence of other injuries

Testing For Meningitis

With the patient supine, place your hand behind her neck and bring the head forward to the chest. In meningitis, the patient responds by flexing hips and knees.

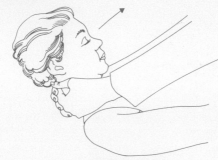

Brudzinski's sign

With the patient supine, flex one leg at the hip and knee to 90° and then straighten the knee. In meningitis, the patient experiences pain because of meningeal and spinal root inflammation.

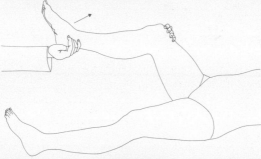

Kernig's sign

Disorders Affecting Arterial or Cerebrospinal Fluid Circulation

TRANSIENT ISCHEMIC ATTACK

Chief complaint
• *Motor disturbances*: depends on location of ataxia; dizziness; falling; weakness
• *Sensory deviations*: numbness, depending on location of affected artery; paresthesias; double vision; fleeting monocular blindness
• *Altered level of consciousness*: drowsiness, giddiness, decreased level of consciousness

History
• Higher incidence in black men over age 50
• Symptoms include atherosclerosis, transient neurologic deficit lasting seconds to no more than 24 hours; hypertension.

Physical examination
• Normal neurologic examination between episodes

ARTERIOVENOUS MALFORMATION

Chief complaint
• *Headache*: migraine on side of malformation; accompanied by vomiting
• *Motor disturbances*: signs of increased intracranial pressure, depending on area of malformation; paresis and cerebrovascular accident from rupture

• *Seizures*: general, focal, or jacksonian; may be first sign of rupture resulting from ischemia
• *Sensory deviations*: visual disturbances; sensory loss depending on area involved; symptoms same as hemorrhage from cerebrovascular accident
• *Altered level of consciousness*: dementia resulting from brief ischemia

History
• Patient may complain of swishing sensation in head; sudden "stroke" in young patients

Physical examination
• Pulsating exophthalmos from ocular pressure; papilledema; retinal hemorrhage if carotid artery bleeds into cavernous sinus; hydrocephalus if membrane causes pressure on aqueduct of Sylvius; bruits over lesion, which disappear with pressure over ipsilateral carotid artery

CEREBROVASCULAR ACCIDENT

Chief complaint
• *Headache/pain*: present, when affecting carotid artery
• *Motor disturbances*: when affecting middle cerebral artery, aphasia, dysphasia, contralateral

Continued

Disorders Affecting Arterial or Cerebrospinal Fluid Circulation
Continued

CEREBROVASCULAR
ACCIDENT *Continued*

hemiparesis or hemiplegia; when affecting carotid artery, weakness, contralateral paralysis or paresis; when affecting vertebral and basilar arteries, contralateral weakness, diplopia, poor coordination, dysphagia, ataxia; when affecting anterior cerebral artery, weakness, loss of coordination, impaired motor function, incontinence; when affecting posterior cerebral artery, contralateral hemiplegia
• *Sensory deviations*: when affecting middle cerebral artery, pain and tenderness in affected arm or leg, numbness, tingling; when affecting carotid artery, numbness and sensory changes on opposite side, visual disturbances on same side, transient blindness; when affecting vertebral and basilar arteries, visual field cut, numbness around lips and mouth, dizziness, blindness, deafness; when affecting anterior cerebral artery, numbness of lower leg or foot, impaired vision; when affecting posterior cerebral artery, visual field cut, pain and temperature impairment, cortical blindness
• *Altered level of consciousness*: when affecting middle cerebral ar-

tery, altered level progressing to coma; when affecting carotid artery, mental confusion, poor memory; when affecting vertebral and basilar arteries, amnesia, confusion, loss of consciousness; when affecting anterior cerebral artery, confusion, personality changes; when affecting posterior cerebral artery, coma
History
• Precipitating factors include atrial fibrillation, subacute bacterial endocarditis, recent heart valve surgery, lung abscess, tuberculosis, air embolism during abortion, pulmonary trauma, surgery, thrombophlebitis, transient ischemic attack, diabetes mellitus, gout, arteriosclerosis, intracerebral tumors, trauma.
Physical examination
• Labored breathing; rapid pulse rate; fever; nuchal rigidity; evidence of emboli to arms, legs, and intestines and other organs, such as spleen, kidneys, or lungs
• When affecting carotid artery, bruits over artery

CEREBRAL ANEURYSM AND INTRACEREBRAL OR SUBARACHNOID HEMORRHAGE

Chief complaint
• *Headache:* sudden, severe
Continued

NEUROLOGIC DISORDERS

Disorders Affecting Arterial or Cerebrospinal Fluid Circulation
Continued

CEREBRAL ANEURYSM AND INTRACEREBRAL OR SUB-ARACHNOID HEMORRHAGE
Continued

headache, with nausea and projectile vomiting
● *Motor disturbances*: depends on site of aneurysm and degree of bleeding or ischemia; hemiparesis; aphasia; ataxia; vertigo; syncope; facial weakness
● *Seizures*: focal or generalized, depending on area of hemorrhage
● *Sensory deviations*: visual impairment with pressure on optic nerve or chiasm; double vision with third, fourth, and fifth cranial nerve compression
● *Altered level of consciousness*: stupor to coma, irritability

History
● Hemorrhage initiates symptoms.
● Precipitating factors include hypertension, oral contraceptives, A-V malformations, family history.

Physical examination
● Temperature may reach 102° F. (38.9° C.) or higher; irregular respirations, dilated and fixed pupils, papilledema, retinal hemorrhage, bilateral Babinski's reflex early after rupture, positive Brudzinski's and Kernig's signs, nuchal rigidity, signs of increased intracranial pressure, blood in cerebrospinal fluid

EPIDURAL (acute) AND SUBDURAL (acute and chronic) HEMATOMAS

Chief complaint
● *Motor disturbances*: hemiplegia or facial weakness on opposite or same side as hematoma; hemiparesis
● *Seizures*: generalized
● *Altered level of consciousness*: irritability, mental confusion, and progressively decreasing level of consciousness; with chronic form, severe intellectual impairment

History
● Signs occur when hematoma has grown large enough to compromise circulation to the brain (increased intracranial pressure).
● With acute form, complaints rapidly develop (within 48 hours).
● With chronic form, complaints develop more slowly (within a few days to weeks).
● Not all lesions cause signs of increased intracranial pressure (especially chronic).

Physical examination
● Positive Babinski's reflex
● Signs of increased intracranial pressure
● Epidural hematomas cause a rapid rise in intracranial pressure and should be treated as a surgical emergency.

Recognizing Stages of Cerebrovascular Disease

If you know or suspect that your patient has cerebrovascular disease, you can assess his condition according to the onset and severity of his symptoms. Use the following stages of cerebrovascular disease as a guide.

For convenience, we've presented each stage in order from least severe to most severe. Your patient may progressively experience each stage or he may experience only one or two of them.

Premonitory phase: Patient experiences generalized warning symptoms which include drowsiness, dizziness, headaches, and occasionally, mental confusion.

Transient ischemic attack (TIA): Neurologic signs and symptoms, caused by temporary interruption of blood supply to the brain, appear and disappear within 24 hours. Most attacks are over within 30 minutes. After an attack, the patient regains complete control of normal functions.

Recurring intermittent neurologic deficit: Neurologic signs and symptoms may last from 12 hours to days or even weeks. The patient will recover completely after the attack, but remains susceptible to relapse. *Important*: Consider a TIA or recurring intermittent neurologic deficit to be a warning sign of stroke from a thrombus or leaking aneurysm.

Progressive stroke: Signs and symptoms evolve slowly over hours or days. At first, the patient shows only a few neurologic signs and symptoms. Then, as his condition worsens, one particular sign or symptom worsens, or new ones appear. He may have such generalized signs and symptoms as headache, vomiting, mental impairment, convulsions, nuchal rigidity, fever, and disorientation. Progressive stroke may be caused by a thrombus extending along an artery to block collateral circulation.

Completed stroke: When the patient's neurologic condition stabilizes, his stroke is considered complete. Neurologic signs and symptoms won't increase or worsen. But they may persist for a long time, and recovery can be slow.

CVA Assessment Aids

- *Angiography*: Helps determine the specific lesion causing a CVA
- *CT scan*: To identify areas of edema, hematomas, infarcts, mass lesions, hydrocephalus
- *Lumbar puncture*: To obtain CSF; bloody or yellow-orange color if stroke is hemorrhagic
- *EEG*: To determine areas of decreased cellular function and potential for seizure activity
- *Brain scan*: To show ischemic area; may be negative for several days after stoke
- *EKG*: To demonstrate heart disease, if present; may be mild ST-T wave changes early after hemorrhagic stroke
- *Cerebral blood flow studies* (currently at only a few large medical centers): To detect deficiencies in cerebral circulation
- *Cerebral-evoked potential testing*: To assess neurologic changes after a stroke
- *Doppler ultrasonography*: To detect arteriovenous disease impairing blood flow
- *Laboratory studies*: To confirm diagnosis; studies include urinalysis, coagulation studies, CBC, serum electrolytes and osmolality, serum glucose, triglycerides, creatinine, and BUN.

CVA Pathophysiology

A cerebrovascular accident (CVA) occurs when there's a decrease in blood supply to a portion of the brain. As you know, interrupted or diminished oxygen supply may cause serious damage to neurons, with possible necrosis, unless normal circulation is restored within a few minutes.

The most common causes of CVA are:
- thrombosis
- embolus
- hemorrhage.

In a thrombotic stroke, the cerebral artery lumen becomes occluded, usually because of atherosclerosis. This is the most common type of cerebrovascular disease, generally occurring in the middle-late years.

An embolism, however, can occur at any age. When an embolus reaches the cerebral vasculature, it may lodge at a narrowed portion of an artery, thereby cutting off circulation. Most susceptible to emboli are patients who have:
- mural thrombi from atherosclerotic or rheumatic heart disease
- thrombi secondary to myocardial infarction
- recently undergone cardiac surgery.

Medications for CVA Patients

Medications that may be routinely given to patients with CVA are:
- *Anticonvulsants:* Dilantin or phenobarbital, to prevent or treat seizures
- *Antihypertensives:* When diastolic pressure's greater than 110 mm Hg or after hypertensive strokes
- *Steroids:* To treat associated cerebral edema
- *Stool softeners*
- *Analgesics:* Codeine for severe headache after hemorrhagic stroke (aspirin may be contraindicated for hemorrhagic patients because it can prolong bleeding time)
- *Vasodilators:* To treat occlusive CVA
- *Anticoagulants or aspirin:* To prevent or treat pulmonary emboli and deep vein thrombosis. (These drugs contraindicated if CVA's cause is hemorrhage.)

CVA Danger Signals

Any of these conditions in CVA patients may indicate a serious, perhaps life-threatening situation:
- Deteriorating level of consciousness
- Respiratory changes iwth blood-gas deterioration
- Blood pressure spikes
- Onset, recurrence, worsening of motor deficits
- Onset, recurrence, worsening of vision difficulties
- Onset, recurrence, worsening of speech problems

CVA Surgery

When the doctor chooses surgery for a CVA patient, he hopes to prevent further strokes, not treat the current stroke. Candidates are usually patients with transient ischemic attacks (TIAs), or with a completed stroke of mild-to-moderate degree. The most common surgical procedures are:

• *Carotid endarterectomy*, in which atherosclerotic plaques that might cause TIAs are removed from the inner arterial wall. The endarterectomy is usually performed at the bifurcation of the artery, where the plaques commonly occur.

Postoperative nursing tips:
—Because heparin is used during the procedure, be sure to observe carefully for postoperative hemorrhage.

—Check speech, level of consciousness, pupillary signs, motor functioning, and superior temporal artery pulse.

• *Microvascular bypass*, a relatively new procedure, may be used to improve intracranial circulation. Candidates may include patients with inaccessible carotid stenosis; vertebrobasilar stenosis or occlusion; or middle cerebral artery stenosis or occlusion. An extracranial vessel, such as the superficial temporal artery, is surgically anastomosed with an intracranial vessel, such as the middle cerebral artery. In this way, collateral circulation is created, bypassing the stenosis or occlusion.

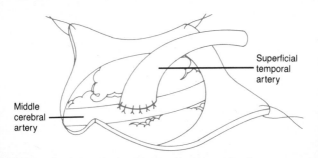

Superficial
temporal
artery

Middle
cerebral
artery

MICROVASCULAR BYPASS

CVA Postoperative Nursing Tips

To care for your CVA patient after he's had surgery:

• Check superficial temporal and carotid artery pulses.

• Check for infection or hemorrhage.

• Monitor blood pressure closely to maintain at optimum preoperative level. Deviations may lead to thrombosis or hemorrhage at the anastomotic site.

• Check neurologic signs for possible deficits. They may indicate an ischemic attack.

• Anticipate aspirin therapy for 4 to 6 weeks to prevent clumping of platelets at the anastomotic site.

• Position the patient so he doesn't lie on the operative side. Doing so may help prevent occlusion.

NEUROLOGIC DISORDERS

Locating Common Communication Disorders

DISORDER/CLINICAL FINDINGS

Broca's aphasia (motor expressive nonfluent)
Patient knows what he wants to say, but has motor impairment
and can't articulate spontaneously. Also patient understands
written or verbal requests but can't repeat words or phrases.

Wernicke's aphasia (sensory receptive/expressive fluent)
Patient articulates spontaneously and well, but uses words in-
appropriately and/or uses neologisms. Also, patient has difficulty understanding written or verbal requests and can't repeat
words or phrases.

Global aphasia
Patient has profound expressive and receptive deficits and can
barely communicate.

Anomia
When given an object, patient can describe its characteristics
(color, size, purpose) but cannot name it.

Apraxia
When asked to speak, patient can't coordinate movement of
lips and tongue. When left alone, he may be able to do so.

Dysarthria
Patient knows what he wants to say, but has motor impairment,
and fails to speak clearly. Also, patient has difficulty swallowing
and chewing.

Perseveration
Patient continually repeats one idea or response.

LOCATION OF LESION

Frontal (posterior)

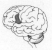

Temporoparietal (anterior)

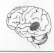

Temporoparietal

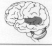

Parietal, subcortical, and/or temporal

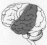

Frontal

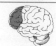

Cerebellar and/or frontal (posterior)

Throughout cerebrum (primarily anterior)

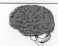

Aphasia

When a patient's brain becomes damaged from a CVA, he may suffer aphasia, which is a loss of power to express or comprehend language. Depending on where the lesion is, aphasia can be of the *expressive* type, in which the patient has difficulty expressing what he thinks, or of the *receptive* type, in which he has trouble understanding what people are telling him.

For example, the patient with expressive aphasia has trouble naming objects and using the correct words to express himself. What's more, he may also have difficulty expressing himself in writing. The patient with receptive aphasia will have trouble reading, following even simple instructions, and recognizing people and things. As a result, his verbal responses may not always be appropriate. Sometimes patients will have a combination of these two types.

Many patients with aphasia recover some of their ability to speak and comprehend during the first several months after a CVA. But even if such spontaneous recovery is very good, progress can be improved if a speech therapist works with the patient. Speech therapy should begin as soon as the patient is physically able. The speech therapist can also give tips to you and the patient's family so you can better communicate with him, as well as suggestions on how to help him.

Ten tips on communicating with the aphasic patient

1. Talk to your patient as an adult; aphasia doesn't mean he has lost his intelligence.
2. Speak slowly and use simple, short sentences along with gestures, when possible.
3. Don't shout; hearing loss is not part of aphasia and shouting will not help the patient understand.
4. Speak to the patient frequently; don't neglect him because he doesn't understand what you say or has trouble communicating—this approach may cause him to feel isolated and he may withdraw into silence.
5. Be honest with your pa-

Continued

Aphasia
Continued

tient; don't pretend you understand if you don't. He may be trying to tell you something important.

6. Remember, your patient may be experiencing extreme frustration as he attempts and fails to perform tasks that were previously routine. Anticipate displays of emotion as he tries to cope with incapacity, and offer him your reassurance as these feelings surface.

7. Avoid the tendency to talk for the patient or frequently supply him with words; have patience with his efforts, slow as they may be.

8. Check whether the patient has auditory comprehension by asking him a question that requires a "no" answer; he's more likely to answer "yes" to all questions. For example, "Did you have soup for breakfast this morning?"

9. Use a set of cards with words such as "bedpan," "thirsty," or "hurt," to help the patient communicate needs and reduce frustration. Encourage him to communicate by writing, if he's able. (Don't use these approaches alone, without efforts to communicate verbally.)

10. Avoid tiring the patient; aphasia gets worse with fatigue or emotional upset.

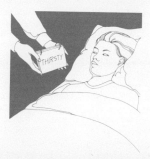

Guide to Headaches

Headaches are one of the most common patient complaints you'll encounter. But are you familiar with the various types of headaches? If you need to know more, study the following chart.

VASCULAR

Possible causes

Intracranial vasoconstriction, followed by extracranial vasodilation of cerebral arteries. May result from use of vasodilators (such as nitrates, alcohol, and histamines), systemic disease, hypoxia, hypertension, head trauma, tumor, or intracranial bleeding

Characteristics

• Signs and symptoms may be aggravated by alcoholic beverages, oral contraceptives, menstruation, stress, and foods containing tyramine.

• *Classic migraine:* occurs unilaterally, primarily in the temporal or frontal area; usually periodic and recurrent; high hereditary incidence; personality factors may contribute

• *Common migraine:* may be unilateral and spreading; gradual onset episodic; high hereditary incidence; signs and symptoms may be relieved by pregnancy; increases with each life crisis

• *Cluster migraine* (histamine headaches): excruciatingly painful, unilateral headaches that occur at the same time each day for a few days. These attacks are followed by remission with no signs or symptoms and then occur weeks, months, or even years later. Cluster migraine headaches are more common in men than in women and are most likely to occur at night.

Signs and symptoms

• *Classic migraine:* transient visual field defects, such as flashing or zigzag lights, followed by severe unilateral pain in temporal or frontal area; transient paralysis; paralysis of an arm or leg; confusion; photophobia; nausea; vomiting; irritability; chills; sweating; constipation

• *Common migraine:* vague psychic disturbances for several hours or days before headache begins; nausea; vomiting; chills; nasal stuffiness; localized or generalized edema; diuresis

• *Cluster migraine:* intense, unilateral throbbing pain beginning high in the nostril and spreading to one side of the forehead, around and behind the eye on the affected side; possibly nasal and ocular lacrimation on this side, reddening of skin, and nasal congestion

MUSCULAR CONTRACTION
(tension)

Possible causes

• Sustained muscle contractions

Continued

Guide to Headaches
Continued

MUSCULAR CONTRACTION
Continued

around the scalp, face, neck, and upper back; vasodilation of associated cranial arteries may contribute to muscle irritability and head pain on the affected side.
Characteristics
• May be unilateral or bilateral; pain frequently occurs in occipital and upper cervical areas and radiates over top of head
• Headaches may be unrelieved for weeks, months, or years.
• Fleeting but recurrent headaches
• Gradual onset
• May be associated with depression or anxiety
Signs and symptoms
• Dull, persistent ache
• Tender spots on head and neck
• Dizziness, tinnitus, lacrimation
• Feelings of tightness around the head (hatband sensation), pressure, or fullness; pain may be localized or vary in location as well as intensity
• Nausea and vomiting

TRACTION AND INFLAMMATORY

Possible causes
• *Traction:* direct nerve pressure from disease or injury; for example, blood clot, brain tumor, or abscess
• *Inflammatory:* primary inflammation that affects specific structures in the head; for example, the meninges (meningitis), sinuses (sinusitis), cranial nerves (trigeminal or glossopharyngeal neuralgia)
Characteristics
• Headaches follow injury or disease (secondary sign)
• May lead to irreversible complications
• Exposure to cold may precipitate or aggravate headache
• *Trigeminal neuralgia* (tic douloureux): unilateral headache involves the face and head and occurs in episodes lasting from 15 seconds to 4 minutes; most common in women over age 40
• *Glossopharyngeal neuralgia:* onset occurs at back of throat and tongue, spreading upward and outward to ears
Signs and symptoms
• Variable, depending on the underlying cause; in most cases, sudden onset, possibly fever (either accompanying the headache or following it)
• Possible convulsions
• Visual disturbances
• Mental changes (apathy, euphoria, inattentiveness)
• Muscle weakness and paresthesia
• Pain ranging from mild and intermittent to sharp and stabbing

Continued

NEUROLOGIC DISORDERS

Guide to Headaches
Continued

TRACTION AND INFLAMMA-
TORY
Continued

• Nausea and vomiting
• *Tumor:* severe pain when patient awakens

• *Intracranial bleeding:* paresthesias and muscle weakness
• *Tic douloureux:* aching, burning,
stabbing pain, usually unilateral
• *Trigeminal or glossopharyngeal
neuralgia:* sharp, stabbing facial
pain in one or more of the nerve's
three branches; may be triggered by
cold winds, touching, or talking

Treating a Headache: Some Alternatives

What's the best way to manage
your patient's headache? That depends on the type of headache,
its severity, and the patient's age
and condition.
Drugs
Analgesics may provide symptomatic relief. A muscle relaxant may
help relieve a muscle tension
headache. For migraine headaches, ergotamine tartrate alone
or combined with caffeinic beverages may be the most effective
treatment. Although migraine
headaches can't be prevented,
methysergide maleate (Sansert*)
can help reduce their frequency
and intensity. During acute headache attacks, your patient may
find that a tranquilizer or an anti-
depressant helps relieve his
symptoms.

Alternative pain relief measures
Familiarize your patient with alternative pain relief measures to
help prevent or treat his headache. *Remember:* Before administering any type of medication or
treatment, try to identify the
cause of your patient's headaches. As you take his history,
look for clues of excessive stress.
    Also check for other causes of
the headaches, such as recent or
previous head trauma, high blood
pressure, arthritis, or allergies.
Refer your patient to a doctor for
further evaluation and treatment.
    Other pain-relieving measures
include:
• simple relaxation techniques
• highly structured relaxation
methods
• acupuncture or acupressure
• electrical stimulation
• biofeedback.

*Available in both the United States and Canada

Most Common Sites of Cerebral Aneurysms

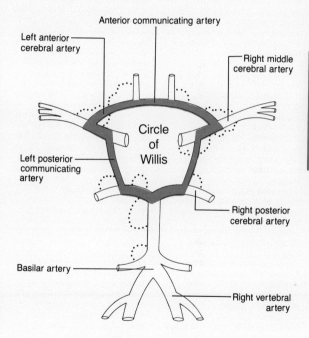

NEUROLOGIC DISORDERS

Note: Dotted lines indicate aneurysm sites

Identifying Major Threats of Aneurysms

The patient with a ruptured cerebral aneurysm faces three major threats, as outlined below:

The initial bleed. As blood escapes into the brain tissue, increased intracranial pressure may cause brain tissue to shift downward, displacing brain stem structures and possibly cutting off blood supply to supporting vital tissues.

Rebleeding. After the leakage of 10 to 20 ml of blood, bleeding usually stops and a clot seals over the rupture, reinforcing the aneurysm for 7 to 10 days. However, around the 7th day, the clot begins to undergo the natural lytic process, and the chances of rebleeding from the same site rise.

If the patient's aneurysm rebleeds, he's faced with the same dangers he faced during the inital bleed.

Vasospasm. When vasospasm occurs, it indicates constriction of intracranial blood vessels from smooth muscle contraction. Vasospasm's cause is unknown, but it usually occurs in the vessel adjacent to the ruptured aneurysm. It may spread through the major vessels at the base of the brain. This results in ischemia and possible infarction of involved areas, which will alter the functions controlled by those areas.

Caution: Watch for the symptoms of vasospasm shortly after the patient's initial bleed and also after surgical repair of the aneurysm. Call the doctor immediately if your patient develops hemiparesis, visual disturbances, seizures, or decreasing level of consciousness.

Grading Aneurysms

The severity of symptoms from ruptured cerebral aneurysm varies with the size and profuseness of the bleed. Here are descriptive categories:
• Grade I—mild bleed; alert, minimal headache, slight nuchal rigidity, no neurologic deficit
• Grade II—mild bleed; alert; mild-to-severe headache, nuchal rigidity; minimal neurologic deficit

as a third nerve palsy
• Grade III—moderate bleed; drowsy or confused; nuchal rigidity; may have mild focal deficit
• Grade IV—moderate or severe bleed; stuporous; nuchal rigidity; may have mild-to-severe hemiparesis
• Grade V—severe bleed; in deep coma; decerebrate movements; possibly moribund.

Surgery for Cerebral Aneurysms

For aneurysm patients, surgical treatment is the only sure method to prevent a rebleed. Here are the three procedures most commonly used:

1

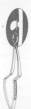

Figure 1 shows a clip applied to the neck of an aneurysm. The clip may be one of several types, all of which are designed to exclude the defective area from circulation. Later, the arterial wall repairs itself, and the necrotic tissue detaches and is reabsorbed.

2

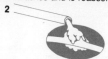

Figure 2 illustrates a procedure the doctor may use when an aneurysm site's inaccessible. The surgeon reinforces the aneurysm wall by wrapping it with:
• muscle, fascia, or other biologic material
• muslin or other types of cloth
• acrylic resins or other types of plastic.

3

Figure 3 shows placement of a carotid artery clamp, used to reduce blood pressure and flow within aneurysms of the internal carotid artery, or other aneurysms inaccessible to direct attack.

Following surgery, the doctor gradually tightens the clamp over a period of several days, thereby allowing time for collateral circulation to compensate for the reduced blood flow.

In caring for the patient at this stage of treatment, you should:
• Document how far the clamp is closed.
• Check neurologic signs every 5 to 10 minutes each time the clamp is tightened.
• Observe for weakness on contralateral side, and dysphasia (if left carotid clamped).
• Record temporal pulses with each neurologic check.
• Be sure handles to clamp are sterile and at bedside.
• Observe for possible infection; inspect dressing frequently.
• Position patient carefully to avoid pressure on dressing.

Hazards for Aneurysm Patients

Pulmonary emboli threaten any immobilized patient, but especially the patient with a ruptured cerebral aneurysm. He'll be particularly susceptible if he's getting an antifibrinolytic drug like aminocaproic acid (Amicar) to delay clot lysis. Because the patient's activity is restricted, fit him with elastic stockings or Ace bandages immediately after admission and use them until activity is resumed.

Should emboli occur despite all precautions, they usually bring chest pains, shortness of breath, dusky color, low PO_2 levels, tachycardia, fever, and a change in the patient's sensorium. Watch for any of these—changes may be subtle—and report them at once.

Treatment of emboli is usually through anticoagulant therapy, which is particularly dangerous for the aneurysm patient because it increases the chances of rebleeding at the aneurysm site.

Be sure to:
● Observe for bleeding tendencies by checking all stool, emesis, and sputum for blood.
● Report at once any change in neurologic status.
● Maintain pulmonary hygiene and monitor arterial blood gas measurements to ensure adequate oxygenation.

Hydrocephalus, an engorgement of cerebrospinal fluid (CSF) in the cerebral ventricles, may follow a subarachnoid hemorrhage.

Special Consideration

Remember these important points when caring for a patient with a cerebral aneurysm rupture:
● Suspect this condition in a patient with neck stiffness, back and leg pain, fever, restlessness, irritability, occasional seizures, and blurred vision. These symptoms result from meningeal irritations caused by bleeding.
● Be sure to establish and maintain an open airway, monitor neurologic status and record your findings, and provide bed rest with limited activity.
● Be aware that surgical treatment of a cerebral aneurysm is the only way to prevent a rebleed.
● Fit your patient with elastic stockings or Ace bandages immediately after admission, and apply them until he resumes activities. Remember, a patient with a cerebral aneurysm is particularly susceptible to pulmonary embolism.
● Observe your patient for these life-threatening problems: rebleeding from the same site, vasospasm, pulmonary embolism, and hydrocephalus.

Testing for Metabolic and Toxic Disorders

Metabolic disorders
Blood tests
• Detect rising levels of liver enzymes and ammonia in hepatic encephalopathy and Reye's syndrome.
• Detect rising blood urea nitrogen and creatinine levels in uremic encephalopathy.
• Show depressed oxyhemoglobin levels and increased carboxyhemoglobin saturation in carbon monoxide poisoning.

Radiologic tests
• Skull X-rays and CT scan can demonstrate small or "absent" ventricles caused by cerebral edema in Reye's syndrome or other conditions such as hepatic or uremic encephalopathy. CT scan also demonstrates cerebral atrophy and helps rule out other conditions.

Electroencephalography
• Reveals a slow pattern in hypoxic, hepatic, and uremic encephalopathy and may indicate a seizure tendency.

Toxic disorders
Blood and urine screening
• Acidification and illumination of a urine sample detect coproporphyrin, a product of poor heme synthesis in lead poisoning.
• Urinalysis can detect all narcotics and can quantify arsenic, mercury, amphetamines, and most narcotics.
• Serum analysis can detect barbiturates, alcohol (ethanol), and manganese.

Special tests
• Skeletal X-rays reveal lead lines in long bones of children, helping confirm chronic lead poisoning.
• CT scan may detect degenerative or hemorrhagic cerebral lesions in heavy metal poisoning, alcoholism, and Wernicke-Korsakoff syndrome.
• EEG reveals a slow pattern in heavy metal poisoning and in barbiturate and narcotic abuse.
• In botulism, EMG shows diminished muscle action potential after one supramaximal nerve stimulus.

NEUROLOGIC DISORDERS

Understanding Metabolic and Toxic Disorders

METABOLIC DISORDERS

HYPOXIC ENCEPHALOPATHY

Causes
Carbon monoxide poisoning, congestive heart failure, coronary artery disease, suffocation, respiratory failure
Pathophysiologic mechanisms
Hypoxia causes cessation of aerobic metabolism, which sustains Krebs cycle and electron transport. Neurons catabolize to compensate for loss of their intrinsic energy source but undergo irreversible damage. Accumulated catabolic products fill interstitial tissue, leading to parenchymal damage.
Signs and symptoms
Confusion, stupor, or coma

HEPATIC ENCEPHALOPATHY

Causes
Hepatitis, cirrhosis, portalsystemic shunt
Pathophysiologic mechanisms
Ammonia, formed in the bowel, fails to be converted to urea in the liver. It enters systemic circulation, reaches the brain, and interferes with cerebral metabolism.
Signs and symptoms
Prodromal stage: disorientation, forgetfulness, slurred speech, slight tremor. *Impending stage:* tremor, asterixis, lethargy, apraxia. *Stuporous stage:* hyperventilation, agitation. *Comatose stage:* hyperactive reflexes, positive Babinski's sign, fetor hepaticus, coma

UREMIC ENCEPHALOPATHY

Causes
Acute and chronic renal failure, dialysis, renal transplantation
Pathophysiologic mechanisms
Excretion of nitrogenous wastes and fluid and electrolyte balance are disrupted. Metabolic acidosis, hypocalcemia, hyperphosphatemia, hypernatremia, hyperkalemia, and increased blood urea nitrogen (BUN) and creatinine levels cause CNS and peripheral nerve irritation.
Signs and symptoms
Apathy, fatigue, inattention, irritability, clouded sensorium, hallucinations, muscle twitching, seizures, Kussmaul's and Cheyne-Stokes respirations, coma

REYE'S SYNDROME

Causes
Cause unknown but follows acute viral infection, such as influenza type B and varicella, in children and adolescents
Pathophysiologic mechanisms
Disruption of urea cycle causes hyperammonemia, hypoglycemia, and increased serum fatty acids
Continued

Understanding Metabolic and Toxic Disorders
Continued

METABOLIC DISORDERS
Continued

REYE'S SYNDROME
Continued

with subsequent alteration in cerebral metabolism. Fatty infiltration of renal tubules and liver occurs. Encephalopathy results from massive cerebral edema and hepatic dysfunction.

Signs and symptoms
Stage I: vomiting, lethargy, hepatic dysfunction. *Stage II:* disorientation, delirium, agitation, hyperventilation, hyperactive reflexes, hepatic dysfunction. *Stage III:* coma, decorticate posturing, hepatic dysfunction. *Stage IV:* deepening coma, decerebrate rigidity, loss of vestibuloocular reflexes, large fixed pupils, increasing hepatic dysfunction. *Stage V:* seizures, absent deep tendon reflexes, respiratory arrest, flaccidity.

TOXIC DISORDERS

ALCOHOLISM

Causes
Exact cause unknown, but family background apparently contributes
Pathophysiologic mechanisms
Alcohol depresses subcortical structures that normally regulate cerebrocortical activity, producing initial excitability of cerebral cortex. Spinal motor neurons initially escape inhibition from higher centers, causing hyperactive tendon reflexes. With increasing amounts of alcohol, depressant action spreads to cerebral cortex, brain stem, and spinal neurons.
Signs and symptoms
Intoxication: confusion, stupor, inattentiveness, memory lapses, aggressive behavior.
After abstinence: nervousness, irritability, diaphoresis, nausea, vomiting; all temporarily relieved by drinking alcohol. Abrupt withdrawal after prolonged or massive use causes delirium tremens (DTs)

WERNICKE-KORSAKOFF SYNDROME

Causes
Thiamine deficiency usually stemming from chronic alcohol abuse
Pathophysiologic mechanisms
Thiamine deficiency impairs production of coenzymes necessary for CNS energy production. Necrosis and vascular changes occur in the hypothalamus, thalamus, and brain stem. Cerebellar atrophy also results.
Signs and symptoms
Confusion, apathy, listlessness, memory loss, inattentiveness, ocular nerve paralysis, ataxia
Continued

NEUROLOGIC DISORDERS

Understanding Metabolic and Toxic Disorders
Continued

TOXIC DISORDERS *Continued*

NARCOTIC ANALGESIC ABUSE

Causes
Exact cause unknown, but inability to cope with stress and frustration, desire for immediate gratification, insecurity, and low self-esteem contribute

Pathophysiologic mechanisms
Analgesics bind with opiate receptors at many CNS sites, altering release of acetylcholine, norepinephrine, substance P, and dopamine—thereby inhibiting neurotransmission. Physical and psychological dependence occur.

Signs and symptoms
Acute: hypotension, bradycardia, pinpoint pupils, coma, respiratory depression. *Withdrawal:* diaphoresis, nausea, vomiting, diarrhea, insomnia, dilated pupils, runny nose and tearing eyes, anorexia, chills, fever, persistent back and abdominal pain, tachycardia, increased blood pressure and respiratory rate, spontaneous orgasm

BARBITURATE ABUSE

Causes
Exact cause unknown, but inability to cope with stress and frustration, desire for immediate gratification, insecurity, and low self-esteem contribute

Pathophysiologic mechanisms
Barbiturates cause CNS depression by decreasing excitability of nerve cells, possibly through increased postsynaptic inhibition of neurotransmission. Physical and psychological dependence can occur.

Signs and symptoms
Acute: progressive CNS and respiratory depression. *Chronic:* slurred speech, poor coordination, decreased mental alertness, memory loss, depressed pulse rate and deep tendon reflexes, nystagmus, diplopia, hypotension, dehydration. *Withdrawal:* nervousness, seizures, irritability, orthostatic hypotension, tachycardia, hallucinations, insomnia

AMPHETAMINE ABUSE

Causes
Exact cause unknown, but inability to cope with stress and frustration, desire for immediate gratification, insecurity, and low self-esteem contribute

Pathophysiologic mechanisms
Amphetamines facilitate CNS neurotransmission by increasing the release of the neurotransmitters dopamine, epinephrine, and 5-HT from storage sites in the

Continued

Understanding Metabolic and Toxic Disorders
Continued

TOXIC DISORDERS *Continued*

AMPHETAMINE ABUSE
Continued

nerve terminals. Neurologic and metabolic stimulation and appetite depression result. Psychological dependence can occur.

Signs and symptoms
Acute: anxiety, hyperactivity, irritability, insomnia, muscle tension, aggressive or violent behavior, paranoia, psychosis, fever, palpitations, hypertension or hypotension, tachycardia, convulsions, abdominal pain.
Withdrawal: depression, overwhelming fatigue

LEAD POISONING

Causes
Ingestion of lead-based paint chips or inhalation of lead containing dust or fumes. More common in children than adults

Pathophysiologic mechanisms
Accumulation of lead in the brain causes massive swelling and herniation of cerebellum and temporal lobes, hemorrhage and ischemia in cerebrum and cerebellum, and deposits of protein and mononuclear inflammatory cells around many small blood vessels.

Signs and symptoms
Vomiting, behavior changes, and, at times, seizures, mental deterioration, irritability, and coma

ARSENIC POISONING

Causes
Inhalation of arsenic-containing insecticides or paint, metal, or enamel fumes

Pathophysiologic mechanisms
Arsenic forms bonds with sulfhydryl radicals, which appear in peripheral nerve axons and capillary endothelial cells in cerebral tissue and are necessary for cellular metabolism. It causes polyneuropathy and hemorrhagic leukoencephalopathy.

Signs and symptoms
Headache, drowsiness, confusion, delirium, seizures, and, in chronic poisoning, weakness, muscle aches, chills, fever, mucosal irritation

MERCURY POISONING

Causes
Chronic inhalation or ingestion of mercury-containing compounds found in work environment or contaminated water or food

Pathophysiologic mechanisms
Mercury inactivates sulfhydryl enzymes and interferes with cellular metabolism. It causes neuronal
Continued

NEUROLOGIC DISORDERS

Understanding Metabolic and Toxic Disorders
Continued

NEUROLOGIC DISORDERS

TOXIC DISORDERS *Continued*

MERCURY POISONING
Continued

of the granular layer of the cerebellar cortex.
Signs and symptoms
Weakness, fatigue, depression, lethargy, irritability, confusion, ataxia, dysarthria, and tremors of the extremities, tongue, and lips

MANGANESE POISONING

Causes
Chronic inhalation or ingestion of manganese particles during ore mining or processing
Pathophysiologic mechanisms
Chronic poisoning interferes with neurobiochemical pathways to cause neuronal loss and gliosis of the basal ganglia, resulting in extrapyramidal-like symptoms.
Signs and symptoms
Progressive weakness, fatigue, confusion, hallucinations, drooling, hand tremors, limb stiffness, faint and dysarthric speech, gross rhythmic movement of trunk and head, retropulsive and propulsive gait

TETANUS

Causes
Contamination of wound or burn

by soil, dust, or animal excreta containing *Clostridium tetani*
Pathophysiologic mechanisms
Tetanus exotoxin is thought to suppress spinal and brain stem neurons by blocking postsynaptic inhibition, thereby allowing afferent stimuli to produce an exaggerated response. Reciprocal innervation is also abolished, producing muscle spasm.
Signs and symptoms
Localized: spasm, increased muscle tone near wound. *Systemic:* marked muscle hypertonicity, hyperactive deep tendon reflexes, tachycardia, diaphoresis, low-grade fever, painful and involuntary muscle contractions, trismus (lockjaw), risus sardonicus

BOTULISM

Causes
Ingestion of food contaminated by *Clostridium botulinum*
Pathophysiologic mechanisms
Botulism exotoxin affects the presynaptic endings of the neuromuscular junction, interfering with release of acetylcholine, thus disturbing muscle innervation.
Signs and symptoms
Blurred vision, dysarthria, dysphagia, and other cranial nerve
Continued

Understanding Metabolic and Toxic Disorders
Continued

TOXIC DISORDERS *Continued*

BOTULISM
Continued

impairment followed by descending weakness or paralysis in extremities and trunk dyspnea and respiratory arrest

DIPHTHERIA

Causes
Inhalation or cutaneous contact with

Corynebacterium diphtheriae
Pathophysiologic mechanisms
Formation and absorption of an exotoxin causes cranial nerve and peripheral paralysis by disrupting protein synthesis
Signs and symptoms
Fever, dyspnea, nasal voice, dysphagia, blurred vision, ascending paralysis, respiratory failure, cardiomyopathy

Examples of Effects of Toxins on Neurotransmission

Toxins interfere with neurotransmission by mimicking the actions of neurotransmitter chemicals or by competing with these chemicals for binding sites on the cell membrane.
Impaired acetylcholine release
Normally, the neuron releases the neurotransmitter acetylcholine into the synaptic cleft to complete transmission of a nerve impulse. However, the botulism toxin blocks the release of acetylcholine from the synaptic vesicles
Impaired acetylcholine binding
To accomplish cell depolarization, receptor sites on the muscle membrane take up acetylcholine. However, the neuromuscular blocking agent curare and its medicinal forms, such as pancuronium, compete with acetylcholine for receptor sites, blocking depolarization.
Postsynaptic inhibition
In normal postsynaptic inhibition, the activation of inhibitory fibers diminishes the excitatory response of the neuron. However, the tetanus toxin blocks these inhibitory fibers, causing hyperexcitability of the neuron.

Distinguishing Neuroinfective Diseases

NEUROLOGIC DISORDERS

BACTERIAL

MENINGITIS

Description
Meningeal infection
Cause
Neonates: gram-negative bacilli or anaerobic streptococci
Children: *Hemophilus influenzae*
Adults: *Neisseria meningitidis* or *Streptococcus pneumoniae*

ENCEPHALITIS

Description
Brain parenchymal infection
Cause
Secondary to bacterial meningitis; injury resulting in invasion by clostridia (anaerobic) or staphylococci (aerobic)

BRAIN ABSCESS

Description
Free or encapsulated pus in brain parenchyma
Cause
Secondary to direct invasion (meningeal, ear, sinus, scalp, or bone infection) or blood-borne (distant infection); anaerobes predominate

SUBDURAL EMPYEMA

Description
Pus between dura mater and arachnoid membrane
Cause
Secondary to paranasal sinus or middle-ear infection

CEREBRAL EPIDURAL ABSCESS

Description
Pus in epidural space of brain
Cause
Secondary to head, face, bone, or paranasal sinus infection

SPINAL EPIDURAL ABSCESS

Description
Pus in epidural space of spinal cord
Cause
Secondary to vertebral body infection; metastatic spread from bacteremia

Continued

Distinguishing Neuroinfective Diseases
Continued

BACTERIAL
Continued

NEUROSYPHILIS

Description
Meningeal infection; occasional extension into brain parenchyma
Cause
Treponema pallidum

VIRAL

MENINGITIS

Description
Meningeal infection
Cause
Various viruses

ENCEPHALITIS

Description
Brain parenchymal infection
Cause
Frequent progression of viral meningitis; may be very severe

HERPES ZOSTER (shingles)

Description
Infection of ganglia and innervation area
Cause
Varicella virus

POLIOMYELITIS

Description
Infection involving anterior horn of the gray matter in the spinal cord or medulla
Cause
Poliovirus

RABIES

Description
Acute central nervous system (CNS) infection
Cause
Rabies virus in saliva of infected host

REYE'S SYNDROME

Description
Acute encephalopathy (brain swelling, fatty infiltration, and liver dysfunction)
Cause
Possible complication of viral infections treated with aspirin

Continued

NEUROLOGIC DISORDERS

Distinguishing Neuroinfective Diseases
Continued

VIRAL
Continued

CREUTZFELDT-JAKOB DISEASE

Description
Encephalopathy with dementia and degeneration of pyramidal and extrapyramidal systems; rare, always fatal
Cause
Slow virus; can be transmitted by experimental animals or contaminated surgical instruments or corneal grafts

SUBACUTE SCLEROSING PANENCEPHALITIS

Description
Subacute encephalitis with white matter deterioration and demyelination
Cause
Defective measles virus

PROGRESSIVE MULTIFOCAL LEUKOENCEPHALOPATHY

Description
CNS demyelination; rare
Cause
Opportunistic papovavirus infection in compromised patient

Major Pathogens

• **Bacteria** such as *Clostridium, Escherichia coli, Hemophilus influenzae, Klebsiella, Neisseria meningitidis, Proteus, Pseudomonas, Staphylococcus aureus, Streptococcus*, Groups A and B
• **Fungi** such as *Actinomyces israelii, Aspergillus fumigatus, Blastomyces dermatitidis, Candida albicans, Histoplasma capsulatum*
• **Parasites** such as *Entamoeba histolytica, Schistosoma haematobium, Schistosoma japonicum, Schistosoma mansoni, Taenia echinococcus, Taenia solium, Toxoplasma gondii, Trichinella spiralis*
• **Viruses** such as Adenoviruses, Enteroviruses, Herpesviruses, Myxoviruses and paramyxoviruses

Diagnostic tests

These tests help diagnose neuroinfective diseases:

Computerized tomography (CT) scan
• May show altered tissue density and increased or displaced vascularity to help identify abscess, calcification, cerebral edema, hydrocephalus, infarction, tumor, middle ear/sinus pus collections
• May use contrast medium for sharper image

Cerebral angiography
• Serves as definitive diagnostic tool for vascular conditions
• Detects and defines space-occupying (even avascular) lesions
• Evaluates vessel lumen for patency, thrombosis, occlusion
• Detects vessel displacement, indicating mass effect from abscess, brain herniation, cerebral edema

X-ray study
• Identifies disease foci
• May show sinus/mastoid disease, pineal shift, signs of chronic elevated intracranial pressure (ICP), gas in abscess cavity

Lumbar puncture
• Helps diagnose CNS infections, especially meningitis
• Gives direct ICP information from CSF pressure readings
• Can identify causative organism through stains and cultures
• Measures protein, glucose, and red and white blood cells through laboratory analysis
• Helps identify causative organism and susceptibility to specific antibiotics through culture and sensitivity tests
• May be contraindicated in meningitis with increased ICP (danger of herniation). Preliminary CT scan advised in suspected abscess

Brain biopsy
• Identifies cause of fungal/parasitic infections
• May be only way of diagnosing some viral infections, such as herpes simplex encephalitis

NEUROLOGIC DISORDERS

Managing Fungal and Parasitic Infections

DISORDER/ORGANISM DIAGNOSIS	TREATMENT
Fungal diseases	
Actinomycosis *(Actinomyces israelii)*. Tissue biopsy for Gram stain (usually reveals causative organism)	Antimicrobial: penicillin, tetracycline (alternative). Steroidal: used with antibiotics
Aspergillosis *(Aspergillus fumigatus)*. Tissue culture preferred, but biopsy not always possible (fungus often infests vital tissues). CSF, blood, or sputum culture (less reliable). Identification difficult *(Aspergillus* is a frequent laboratory contaminant)	Antimicrobial: amphotericin B with surgical excision. Steroidal: contraindicated; enhances tissue invasion and fungus dissemination
Blastomycosis *(Blastomyces dermatitidis)*. Brain biopsy for identification and culture. Ventricular or cisternal fluid analysis	Antimicrobial: amphotericin B. Steroidal: usually avoided
Candidiasis *(Candida albicans* and *C. tropicalis)*. Fungus finding in tissue. Fungus identification in CSF or culture. Culture mandatory (species identification cannot be made from direct smears and *Candida* closely resembles other organisms)	Antimicrobial: amphotericin B alone or combined with 5-fluorocytosine. Steroidal: usually avoided
Coccidioidomycosis *(Coccidioides immitis)*. Pathogen identification in cerebral tissue or CSF. Culture from same source (less reliable). Serologic tests: IgM precipitant (positive in about 90% of acutely ill patients)	Antimicrobial: systemic and intrathecal amphotericin B. Steroidal: usually avoided

Continued

Managing Fungal and Parasitic Infections
Continued

DISORDER/ORGANISM DIAGNOSIS	TREATMENT

Fungal diseases
Continued

Cryptococcosis *(Cryptococcus neo-formans)*. CSF culture (positive in about 95% of infected patients). Analysis of sera and CSF for antigen and antibody	Antimicrobial: combination therapy with amphotericin B, 5-fluorocytosine, and miconazole. Steroidal: avoided
Histoplasmosis *(Histoplasma capsulatum)*. Identification of fungus in tissue (especially bone marrow) or isolation in culture	Antimicrobial: amphotericin B. Steroidal: avoided

Parasitic diseases

Amebiasis *(Entamoeba histolytica)*. Identification of trophozoites in biopsy specimens from lesions or in CSF serologic tests (indirect hemagglutination antibody, complement-fixation, agar gel differentiation, indirect immunofluorescent antibody)	Antimicrobial: emetine hydrochloride, metronidazole, chloroquine, tetracycline, diiodohydroxyquin, diloxanide furoate, dehydroemetine. Steroidal: contraindicated
Cysticercosis *(Taenia solium, porcine tapeworm)*. Identification of parasite in nervous tissue, supported by X-ray and immunologic evidence. CT scan for revealing distinct cysts	Antimicrobial: praziquantel. Steroidal: useful to control inflammatory response

Continued

NEUROLOGIC DISORDERS

Managing Fungal and Parasitic Infections
Continued

DISORDER/ORGANISM DIAGNOSIS	TREATMENT

Parasitic diseases
Continued

Echinococcosis *(Taenia echinococcus,* canine tapeworm). Diagnosis dependent on high index of clinical suspicion. Biopsy contraindicated (contamination may imperil operative outcome). Ancillary tests: intradermal, complement-fixation, immunologic panel	Antimicrobial: surgical removal of central nervous system cyst (uniocular cyst); mebendazole (multiocular cysts). Steroidal: helpful in treating cranial nerve palsies from basilar involvement
Schistosomiasis *(Schistosoma mansoni, S. haematobium, S. japonicum).* Isolation of ova in stool, urine, brain tissue, or spinal axis tissue. Ancillary tests: complement-fixation, circumoral precipitin, and indirect fluorescent antibody; CT scan for localizing lesion	Antimicrobial: niridazole *(Schistosoma haematobium),* oxamniquine *(S. mansoni,* and *S. haematobium),* praziquantel *(S. japonicum).* Steroidal: useful adjunct to antimicrobial therapy
Toxoplasmosis *(Toxoplasma gondii).* Diagnosis reliant on immunologic tests (particularly rising antibody titers by complement-fixation, Sabin-Feldman dye, or indirect fluorescent antibody). Possible brain biopsy for definitive diagnosis	Antimicrobial: combination of sulfadiazine and pyrimethamine. Steroidal: large doses in acute stages to combat intense inflammatory response; taper quickly since steroids may reactivate latent cystic foci
Trichinosis *(Trichinella spiralis).* Larva in blood, CSF, or muscle. Serologic tests (precipitin reaction, indirect fluorescent antibody, complement-fixation, bentonite flocculation, and latex agglutination)	Antimicrobial: thiabendazole. Steroidal: methylprednisolone produces dramatic results

Classifying Brain Tumors

Brain tumors can be classified as malignant or benign, as primary or secondary, by cellular origin, by cellular differentiation, or by location.

Malignant or benign

Brain tumors are either malignant or benign. However, even benign tumors can have devastating effects if they're located in a vital area.

Primary or secondary

Almost 90% of brain tumors are *primary*, arising from CNS tissue. Primary tumors rarely metastasize outside the CNS, but they often infiltrate another area of the CNS. The remaining 10% of brain tumors are *secondary*, metastasizing from the lungs, GI tract, breasts, ovaries, or kidneys.

Cellular origin

Brain tumors arise from *neuroectodermal* or *mesodermal* cells. They can be further divided by *specific cell type.* For example, tumors that arise from astrocyte cells are called astrocytomas.

Cellular differentiation

Grading—a measure of cellular differentiation—takes into account the resemblance of tumor tissue to normal cells. *Grade I* shows well-differentiated cells; *grade II,* moderately differentiated; *grade III,* poorly differentiated; and *grade IV,* very poorly differentiated. Typically, grade III and IV tumors are malignant.

Location

Although this classification doesn't provide information on tumor type or prognosis, it does prove helpful for detecting localizing signs. Supratentorial tumors usually develop in the cerebral hemispheres and occasionally in the corpus callosum. Infratentorial tumors develop in the posterior fossa, cerebellum, cerebellopontine angle, and brain stem.

NEUROLOGIC DISORDERS

Intracranial and Spinal Tumors

EXTRAMEDULLARY SPINAL TUMOR (neurinomas, meningiomas, sarcomas)

Chief complaint
• *Headache/pain:* dull aching and soreness of muscles, mild pain along nerve root
• *Motor disturbances:* spastic weakness of muscles below lesion; with severe compression, loss of bladder and bowel control; atrophy of muscles; paraplegia
• *Sensory deviations:* paresthesias; impairment of proprioception and cutaneous sensation below lesion; with severe compression, loss of sensation below lesion

History
• Most common in young and middle-aged adults
• Predisposing factors include Hodgkin's disease and metastatic carcinoma.
• Symptoms worsened by exertion

Physical examination
• Muscle atrophy and impairment of reflexes, depending on location and extent of injury and amount of time since injury occurred; sensory sparing in some cases; with half the cord compressed, Brown-Séquard syndrome

INTRAMEDULLARY SPINAL TUMOR (gliomas)

Chief complaint
• *Headache/pain:* sharp, tearing, or boring pain, depending on location of tumor; increased by movement and relieved by change of posture
• *Motor disturbances:* weakness in one or both legs, clumsiness, shuffling or spastic gait, incontinence
• *Sensory deviations:* paresthesias occur after pain diminishes; complete sparing of sensation in legs possible

History
• Possible limb heaviness or feeling as though walking on air
• Symptoms worsened by exertion

Physical examination
• Overactive leg reflexes, leg weakness, sensory sparing (loss)

INTRACRANIAL TUMORS (medulloblastoma, meningloma, astrocytoma, acoustic neuroma, oligodendroma)

Chief complaint
• *Headache/pain:* headache; worse in morning; may be accompanied by vomiting
• *Motor disturbances:* motor deficits, depending on location of tumor
• *Seizures:* generalized or local, depending on site of tumor

Continued

Intracranial and Spinal Tumors
Continued

INTRACRANIAL TUMORS
Continued

• *Sensory deviations:* dependent on pressure on cranial or olfactory nerves
• *Altered level of consciousness:* progressive deterioration of intellect; behavior changes possible; decreased level of consciousness with increased intracranial pressure
History
• Medulloblastoma most common in young children
• Meningioma most common in women over age 50
• History of present illness includes progressive deterioration of motor function, increasing frequency and duration of headaches, personality changes
Physical examination
• Signs of increased intracranial pressure: widening pulse pressure and bounding pulse (Cushing's phenomenon), ipsilateral (same side as lesion) pupil dilatation and contralateral (opposite side of lesion) muscle weakness (Weber's syndrome), decreasing level of consciousness, irregular respiratory patterns progressing to respiratory arrest, temperature fluctuation, papilledema, decorticate or decerebrate posturing
• Motor and sensory deficits appropriate to affected area

NEUROLOGIC DISORDERS

Brain Tumors: Site-Specific Symptoms

Brain tumors—both benign and malignant—usually produce signs and symptoms specific to their location. Recognizing these helps you identify tumor site, plan pre- and postoperative treatment, and spot life-threatening complications, such as increasing intracranial pressure and imminent brain herniation.

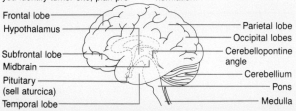

Frontal lobe
Hypothalamus
Subfrontal lobe
Midbrain
Pituitary (sell aturcica)
Temporal lobe
Parietal lobe
Occipital lobes
Cerebellopontine angle
Cerebellium
Pons
Medulla

Tumor Types and Their Locations

TYPE OF TUMOR	COMMON LOCATIONS
Acoustic neuroma	8th cranial nerve, Cerebellopontine angle Cranial nerves adjacent to the 8th (compress 5th, 7th, 9th, and 10th)
Astrocytoma, grades I and II	Cerebral hemispheres (frontal, parietal, and temporal lobes), Cerebellum in children
Astrocytoma, grades III and IV (glioblastoma multiforme)	Frontal lobe Corpus callosum
Craniopharyngioma	Sella turcica
Ependymoma	Ventricular system (especially the 4th ventricle)
Hemangioblastoma	Cerebellum, Cerebral hemispheres, Medulla
Medulloblastoma	Cerebellum, 4th ventricle, Spinal cord
Meningioma	Near the venous sinuses on the convexity of the brain Anterior, posterior fossae floors
Neurofibromatosis (von Recklinghausen's disease)	Throughout the central and peripheral nervous systems
Oligodendroglioma	Cerebral hemispheres (frontal and temporal lobes)
Pituitary adenoma	Sella turcica
Spongioblastoma	Optic nerves

NEUROLOGIC DISORDERS

Guide to Developmental Neurologic Disorders

HYDROCEPHALUS

Chief complaint
● *Motor disturbances:* spastic movements of arms and legs (more severe in legs), increased tendon reflexes
● *Altered level of consciousness:* apathy, lethargy, irritability

History
● Normal head size at birth, increasingly more rapid growth than normal

Physical examination and diagnostic studies
● Head growth exceeds normal by ½″ (1.27 cm) per month; distended scalp veins; full, tense fontanelles; widened cranial sutures; asymmetric appearance of head; setting-sun sign (eyes pushed down in orbit); inability to hold head up; strabismus; cracked-pot sign on skull percussion; high-pitched cry
● Skull transilluminates

Continued

**Normal
Medial view**

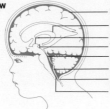

— Subarachnoid space
— Lateral ventricle
— Foramen of Monro
— Third ventricle
— Aqueduct of Sylvius
— Fourth ventricle
— Cisterna magna
— Foramen of Magendie

Hydrocephalus

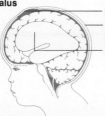

— Bulging fontanel
— Enlarged head circumference
— Enlarged ventricles

Guide to Developmental Neurologic Disorders
Continued

NEUROLOGIC DISORDERS

REYE'S SYNDROME

Chief complaint
• *Motor disturbances:* In stage I, none; in stage II, hyperactive reflexes; in stage III, decorticate rigidity; in stage IV, decerebrate rigidity, large and fixed pupils; in stage V, loss of deep tendon reflexes, flaccidity
• *Seizures:* none, until stage V
• *Altered level of consciousness:* in stage I, lethargy; in stage II, coma; in stage III, deepening coma; in stage IV, deep coma
History
• Acute viral infection 1 to 2 days before onset of symptoms
• Prodromal symptoms include malaise, cough, earache, rhinorrhea, sore throat
Physical examination and diagnostic studies
• Vomiting; hyperventilation or respiratory arrest; hyperactive reflexes; absent deep tendon reflexes; decorticate or decerebrate rigidity; large, fixed pupils; rash
• Serum ammonia level above 300 mg/100 ml, elevated BUN, elevated liver enzymes (SGOT and SGPT), increased intracranial pressure, prolonged prothrombin time, decreased carbon dioxide pressure (arterial blood gases)

SYDENHAM'S CHOREA
(St. Vitus' dance)

Chief complaint
• *Motor disturbances:* sporadic movements of face, trunk, and extremity muscles; incoordination; muscle weakness; facial grimacing; arthritis, arthralgia (growing pains)
• *Altered level of consciousness:* restless, emotional instability
History
• Onset usually between ages 5 and 15
• Symptoms include rheumatic fever, lack of sleep due to involuntary movements, nightmares; progress over 2 weeks
Physical examination and diagnostic studies
• Muscle weakness, facial grimacing, no muscle atrophy or contractures

DOWN'S SYNDROME

Chief complaint
• *Motor disturbances:* generalized muscular hypotonicity; structural, facial abnormalities
• *Altered level of consciousness:* impaired mental capacity
History
• Family history of Down's syndrome
• Most common in infants born to
Continued

Guide to Developmental Neurologic Disorders
Continued

DOWN'S SYNDROME
Continued

mothers over age 35 or in first-born of very young mothers
• Growth and development slower than normal
Physical examination and diagnostic studies
• Gutteral cry; small, round head; flat, occipital, low-set ears; mongoloid slant to eyes; small mouth, with protruding tongue; increased fat pad at nape of neck; short, heavy hands; transverse palmar crease; incomplete Moro's reflex; Brushfield's spots (gray-white specks on iris)

CEREBRAL PALSY (spastic, athetoid, and ataxic forms)

Chief complaint
• *Motor disturbances:* In spastic form, hyperactive deep tendon reflexes, rapid alternating muscle contractions and relaxations; in athetoid form, grimacing, dystonia, wormlike movements, sharp and jerky movements before becoming more severe during stress and disappearing during sleep; in ataxic form, muscle weakness, loss of balance and coordination, especially in arms
• *Seizures:* in spastic form, seizure disorders possible
• *Sensory deviations:* in spastic

form, visual and hearing deficits possible
• *Altered level of consciousness:* in ataxic form, emotional disorders, mental retardation in about 40% of cases
History
• Maternal infection, especially rubella
• Prenatal radiation, anoxia
• Birth difficulties, such as forceps delivery, breech presentation, placenta previa, premature birth
• Infection or trauma during infancy, such as brain infection; head trauma; prolonged anoxia
Physical examination and diagnostic studies
• Underdeveloped affected limbs; hard-to-separate legs; leg crossing, rather than bicycling, when child's lifted from behind; scissors gait; muscle weakness; hyperactive reflexes; contractures; persistent favoring of one hand; nystagmus; dental abnormalities

NEUROFIBROMATOSIS
(von Recklinghausen's disease)

Chief complaint
• *Headache:* pain along nerve distribution
• *Motor disturbances:* rarely any weakness or atrophy
• *Altered level of consciousness:* may occur with brain tumor

Continued

NEUROLOGIC DISORDERS

Guide to Developmental Neurologic Disorders
Continued

NEUROFIBROMATOSIS
Continued

History
• Onset may be anytime from childhood to age 50
• Family history of neurofibromatosis—congenital
• May be accompanied by meningiomas, gliomas of the central nervous system

Physical examination and diagnostic studies
• Multiple tumors under the skin of the scalp, arms, legs, trunk, and cranial nerves; pigmentary lesions, café au lait spots; symptoms similar to brain or spinal tumor, depending on tumor's location; overgrowth of skin and of skull and neck tissue; hypertrophy of face, tongue, arms, and legs; skeletal anomalies; bone cysts
• Cranial nerve abnormalities if affected

PETIT MAL (absence)

Chief complaint
• *Motor disturbances:* myoclonus, automatisms, usually no loss of tone in muscles
• *Seizures:* Petit mal
• *Altered level of consciousness:* brief loss of consciousness characterized by fixed gaze and blank expression; postictal period: immediately followed by alertness

and continued activity

History
• Idiopathic seizure disorder diagnosed usually between ages 4 and 12; onset rare after age 20
• Predisposing factors include birth injury or developmental defect, acute febrile illness

Physical examination and diagnostic studies
• Petit mal triad: myoclonic jerks, automatisms, transient absences
• May only be characterized by brief staring periods with occasional eye blinks

INFANTILE SPASM

Chief complaint
• *Motor disturbances:* sudden dropping of the head and flexing of the arms; clonic movements of the arms and legs; developmental and mental retardation

History
• Usually lasts until 3 or 4 years of age, then possibly changes to generalized seizures

Physical examination and diagnostic studies
• Brief myoclonic jerks involving entire body; lasting a few seconds but may be repeated many times during the day
• Family history of convulsions and neurologic disorders is significant
• EEG changes
• Skull X-ray

Continued

Guide to Developmental Neurologic Disorders
Continued

SPINA BIFIDA

Chief complaint
• *Motor disturbances:* weakness, loss of tendon reflexes in legs, gait disturbances, incontinence
• *Sensory deviations:* impaired cutaneous and proprioceptive senses in legs
History
• May be asymptomatic
• Weakness in legs
• Occasionally associated with bowel and bladder disturbances
• Occasionally associated with syrinomyelia, a condition marked by a fluid-filled cavity (syrinx) within the spinal cord
Physical examination and diagnostic studies
• Palpable defect
• Scoliosis and deformities of feet, usually unilateral
• Radiologic studies of the spine, skull, hips, and lower extremities
• Urinanalysis and urine culture
• BUN and creatinine
• Intravenous pylogram (IVP)

Ventricular Dilation: Hallmark of Hydrocephalus

Medical management
Diagnosis of hydrocephalus can be elusive. Normal-pressure hydrocephalus develops so insidiously that telltale signs are easily overlooked. Even in hydrocephalic infants, an abnormally large head isn't conclusive evidence. Accurate diagnosis, of course, requires a thorough history and physical, but special tests give the best data.
What diagnostic tests reveal
Diagnostic workup for hydrocephalus includes:
Computerized tomography (CT) scan. This test reveals ventricular enlargement in hydrocephalus, helps locate CSF obstruction, identifies intracranial lesions, and shows cortical size and thickness.
Pneumoencephalogram. A possible adjunct to the CT scan, this test pinpoints CSF obstruction and shows ventricular enlargement. In normal-pressure hydrocephalus, the injected air readily fills the ventricles. However, since CSF reabsorption is impeded, movement of air into the cerebral subarachnoid space is slight.
Isotope cisternogram (flow study). This test also pinpoints CSF obstruction and evaluates the rate of CSF reabsorption, helping to distinguish noncommunicating from communicating (particularly normal-pressure).

Types of Spinal Cord Defects

In all types of spina bifida (spinal bifida occulta, meningocele, myelocele, myelomeningocele), the neural tube fails to close in the first month
of gestation. The cause is unknown but may be associated with viruses,
radiation, environmental factors, and genetics.

NEUROLOGIC DISORDERS

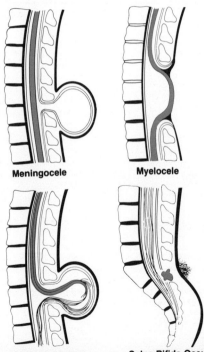

Meningocele

Myelocele

Myelomeningocele

Spina Bifida Occulta

Guide to Head Injuries

As you know, a head injury can have grave, even life-threatening consequences. To prevent complications, proper emergency care is essential. Check patient's airway, respirations, pulse rate, and level of consciousness. Carefully examine patient for other injuries. Pay particular attention to his scalp. *Remember:* Don't move him until he's properly immobilized. Dress any open wounds. Call for medical assistance and stay with patient until help arrives.

Study the chart below to learn about common head injuries.

CEREBRAL CONTUSION
(Bruising of the brain)

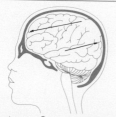

Two types: Coup-countrecoup and acceleration-deceleration
Causes
Blow to the head that bruises the brain directly; for example, from being hit with a blunt instrument. Such a blow drives the brain into the opposite side of the skull, causing more bruising (coup-contrecoup injury). Or, a person's head may be jolted forward, such as in a car accident, causing the brain to slap against the back of the skull. Then, the head stops abruptly, causing the brain to slap against the front of the skull (acceleration-deceleration injury).

Signs and symptoms
• Variable respirations; may range from normal to ataxic, periodic, or rapid
• Rapid pulse
• Drowsiness
• Disorientation and confusion
• Possibly agitation or violent behavior
• Deteriorating level or loss of consciousness
• Usually small, equal, and reactive pupils
• Loss of normal eye movement
• Hemiplegia or, if injury's severe, quadriplegia
• Fever, accompanied by diaphoresis
• Possibly severe scalp wounds
• Decerebrate or decorticate posturing

Continued

NEUROLOGIC INJURIES

Guide to Head Injuries
Continued

SKULL FRACTURE

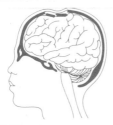

Cause
Blow to the head, possibly resulting from a fight, fall, or motor vehicle accident

Signs and symptoms
• Scalp wounds, abrasions, contusions, lacerations, or avulsions. *Note:* Linear fractures may be insidious and require X-ray confirmation.
• Profuse bleeding, especially with an open fracture
• Persistent, localized headaches
• Changes in respiratory patterns; possibly respiratory distress
• Alterations in level of consciousness; possibly loss of consciousness

• Possible agitation and irritability (with a depressed fracture)
• If bone fragments pierce the dura mater or cerebral cortex, possible subdural, epidural, or intracerebral hemorrhage or hematoma
• With intracranial or intracerebral hemorrhage, hemiparesis, dizziness, convulsions, projectile vomiting, and decreased pulse rate
• With cranial vault fracture, soft-tissue edema in area of fracture
• With basilar fracture, hemorrhaging from the nose, pharynx, or ears; cerebrospinal fluid drainage from the nose or ears; periorbital ecchymosis without a history of eye trauma; supramastoid ecchymosis (Battle's sign); and sometimes bleeding behind the tympanic membrane (hemotatympanum)
• With sphenoidal fracture, optic nerve damage, possibly resulting in blindness
• With temporal fracture, possible unilateral deafness or facial paralysis

Continued

Guide to Head Injuries
Continued

CONCUSSION
(Functional impairment of the brain)

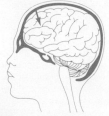

LACERATION
(Penetration of skull and brain by an object)

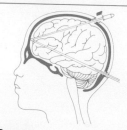

Cause
Blow to the head or face; for example, from a fall, punch, or motor vehicle accident
Signs and symptoms
• Headache
• Dilated pupils
• Restlessness or combative-ness
• Drowsiness
• Vertigo
• Nausea
• Weak pulse
• Unusually rapid or slow breathing
• Brief unconsciousness
• Possible transient amnesia
• Disorientation
• Blurred or double vision (diplopia)

Causes
Blow to the head, such as from a baseball bat, that may fracture the skull and cause bone fragment to tear brain tissue; in other cases, an object, such as a bullet, passing through the skull and brain but not lodging there
Signs and symptoms
• Visible open wound at en-trance and exit sites
• Loss of consciousness
• Bleeding

Continued

Guide to Head Injuries
Continued

PENETRATING SKULL IN-
JURY
(Foreign object in the brain)

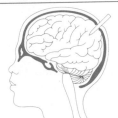

Cause
An object, such as a bullet,
passing through the skull and
lodging in the brain
Signs and symptoms
• Headache
• Bleeding
• Open wound with protrud-
ing object
• Irritability
• Restlessness
• Loss of normal eye move-
ment
• Loss of consciousness

FACIAL FRACTURES

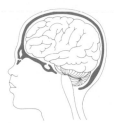

Cause
Direct blow to one of the facial
bones, such as the nasal, mandible, maxillae, or zygomatic,
usually from trauma, such as
from a fall, motor vehicle accident, or contact sport
Signs and symptoms
• Epistaxis, ranging from trick-
ling to full nasal hemorrhage
• Ecchymoses at the affected
site
• Soft-tissue edema
• Head and neck pain
• Facial asymmetry from fracture or soft tissue edema
• Malfunctioning or loss of
function of the affected area
• Possible blood or cerebrospinal fluid drainage from the
nose and ears

Brain Herniation

UNCAL HERNIATION (transtentorial herniation)

Lateral displacement of the brain's medial structures

Cause

Medial portion of temporal lobe slipping across the tentorium into the posterior fossa, caused by an expanding lesion of temporal lobe or a lateral extracerebral lesion

Implications

Exerts pressure on the third cranial nerve and eventually the brain stem

Signs and symptoms

Third nerve palsy (ipsilateral loss of direct reaction to light; ipsilateral ptosis; ipsilateral loss of medial rectus muscle movement; contralateral loss of consensual reaction to light; pupil is small at first, then becomes progressively larger and fixed); upper motor neuron involvement (motor paralysis affecting functionally-related group muscles; jackknife spasticity; hyperactive deep tendon reflexes in involved limbs; loss of cutaneous abdominal and cremasteric reflexes on paralyzed side; presence of Babinski response on paralyzed side; atrophy and fasciculations of involved muscles); loss of doll's eye reflex; decerebrate rigidity; hyperthermia; and other vital function disturbances, such as ataxic respiration pattern

TONSILLAR HERNIATION (medullary cone or cerebellar tonsillar herniation)

Downward displacement of the brain's medial structures

Cause

Cerebellar tonsils pressing on the medulla, caused by an expanding lesion of the hemispheres or a centrally-located extracerebral lesion

Implications

May lead to medullary collapse and death

Signs and symptoms

Altered level of consciousness; nuchal rigidity; upper motor neuron involvement (see above); respiratory changes (frequent sighs and yawns, leading to Cheyne-Stokes pattern and central neurogenic hyperventilation); decorticate posturing, progressing to decerebrate posturing; positive Babinski response; bilateral pupil enlargement; wide fluctuation in body temperature; and medullary collapse (flaccidity, respiration and/or circulatory collapse)

Identifying Lesion Site By Pupillary Signs

When you observe a patient with known or suspected cerebral injury, check for pupillary abnormalities. The type of abnormality is a convenient indicator of the lesion site.

As you know, pupillary constriction responses are controlled by the oculomotor (third cranial) nerve. An increase in intracranial pressure with herniation of brain tissue results in compression of this nerve. And because the *pupilloconstrictor* fibers run along the top of the nerve, they're coimpressed first.

When you examine the pupils, note relative sizes first and then test how the pupils react to light in a darkened room. When the lesion is in one hemisphere, the ipsilateral pupil may remain dilated and unresponsive to light level changes. Eventually, however, both hemispheres are affected by increasing cerebral pressure, and both pupils then remain fixed and dilated.

Supratentorial lesions:
Watch for differences in response to light. Remember, unilateral pupillary dilatation (1) generally occurs ipsilateral to lesion.

In later stage of midbrain compression, the pupils become fixed, and the eyes immobile (2).

Bilateral dilatation (3) indicates upper brain stem damage has already become extremely advanced.

Infratentorial lesions:
With cervical, sympathetic lesion, pupils are unequal, usually fixed. Horner's syndrome may be present. Watch for ptosis; ipsilateral pupillary constriction (4); decreased sweating on same side of face; enophthalmos (sinking in) of eyeball.

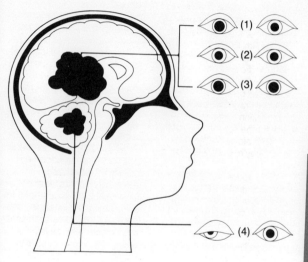

Defining Brain Death

Doctors, lawyers, and legislators have yet to agree on a national definition of brain death. As a result, many states have adopted statutory law definitions of brain death while others have left such definitions to local authorities or individual hospitals. Despite the absence of a uniform definition of brain death, the following criteria are generally accepted as evidence of brain death.

• *Presence of irreversible coma of established cause.* Coma resulting from drug overdose or profound hypothermia must be ruled out.

• *Absence of cerebral function.* Assessment reveals lack of spontaneous movement and no verbal or motor response to any stimulus. Occasionally, spinal reflexes remain intact. A flat (isoelectric) EEG or cessation of cerebral blood flow also provides confirming evidence.

• *Absence of brain stem function.* Assessment reveals no pupillary reaction to light; no corneal, oculocephalic, oculovestibular, oropharyngeal, or tracheal reflexes; no decerebrate or decorticate response to noxious stimuli; and no spontaneous respirations.

These criteria must be met during two or more examinations performed 24 hours apart.

Compassion for the living
Besides aiding in the diagnosis of brain death, your nursing role includes much more. Of course you'll need to provide emotional support for the patient's family. Brain death may be difficult for them to grasp when they see the patient breathing with ventilator assistance and his heartbeat displayed on a monitor. Your human touch and kind explanations can provide much-needed comfort.

Also, if the patient is a potential organ donor, strictly adhere to your institution's donor protocol to help assure successful transplantation.

What Are DSA and MRI?

When the doctor examines your patient with a neurologic emergency, his tentative diagnosis is epidural hematoma. He turns to you and says, "Let's get a DSA on him."

Would you know what to do? What if the doctor ordered "an MRI" instead?

As you probably know, the computerized tomography (CT) scan is the most widely used diagnostic tool for locating an area of injury such as a hematoma. But two new computerized diagnostic tests, in addition to the CT scan, are available: digital subtraction angiography (DSA) and magnetic resonance imaging (MRI)—formerly referred to as nuclear magnetic resonance, or NMR. These tests also produce detailed images of body tissue for evaluating areas of injury or disease. Here's information about DSA and MRI plus comparative information on the CT scan.

DSA: DIGITAL SUBTRACTION ANGIOGRAPHY

What it is

DSA is a type of intravenous arteriography. It combines X-ray methods and a computerized subtraction technique with fluoroscopy for visualization without interference from adjacent structures, such as bone or soft tissue.

How it works

A contrast dye's injected through a catheter threaded into a large vein. As the contrast dye circulates through the arteries, X-rays are taken. The computer then projects the image onto a screen, automatically "subtracting" structures that block a clear view of the arteries and leaving only the vessels being studied.

Benefits

DSA can be performed quickly, even on an outpatient basis, and is an excellent tool for visualizing cerebral blood flow and detecting vascular abnormalities or disruptions, such as aneurysms, tumors, and hematomas. Because the dye's injected into a vein, risk of arterial bleeding is eliminated.

MRI: MAGNETIC RESONANCE IMAGING

What it is

A noninvasive imaging technique that detects structural and biochemical abnormalities by directing magnetic and radio waves at body tissues to determine the nuclear response of a test element—hydrogen.

Continued

NEUROLOGIC INJURIES

What Are DSA and MRI?
Continued

MRI: MAGNETIC RESONANCE
IMAGING
Continued

How it works
MRI uses a resistive magnet that
creates a magnetic field via elec-
tricity. (*Note:* This magnet can affect pacemaker function.) This
magnet causes the body's hydrogen protons to align themselves in
its field. They're then bombarded
with radio frequency signals,
causing them to move out of
alignment. When the radio signal
stops, these energized protons
emit a return signal. A computer
analyzes both this signal and the
time it takes the protons to return
to their original alignment. (The
time and signal vary with each
tissue type.) Eventually, the hydrogen pattern's converted into
an image of body tissue.

Benefits
MRI doesn't use ionizing radiation
(X-rays), so it's safer than CT
scanning or DSA. It doesn't use
contrast dye, either, as DSA (and
sometimes CT) does, so fluid balance problems are eliminated. It
provides greater tissue discrimina-
tion than CT scanning and allows
serial studies to be done safely,
especially in children and pregnant women. In the future, it may
allow visualization of blood flow.

CT: COMPUTERIZED TOMOG-
RAPHY

(Note: Some health-care professionals still refer to this procedure
as computerized axial tomography [CAT].)
A noninvasive X-ray technique
that produces a series of tomo-
grams, translated by a computer
and displayed on an oscilloscope
screen, representing cross-sectional images of various tissue
layers.

How it works
CT scanners use a large circular
X-ray beam in a full circle around
the patient's body or the area
being studied. The computer then
puts the information into cross-
sectional pictures, eliminating the
obstructive shadows that appear
in single X-rays. Contrast dye can
be injected I.V. to enhance tissue
density.

Benefits
CT scanners are widely available
as a diagnostic tool; many hospitals have their own. By discrimi-
nating among minute tissue
density variations, this procedure
can help confirm a diagnosis such
as hematoma or tumor. It may
eliminate the need for more hazardous and painful invasive procedures.

What Happens in Increased Intracranial Pressure

Increased intracranial pressure (ICP) is the pressure exerted within the intact skull by the intracranial volume—about 10% blood, 10% cerebrospinal fluid (CSF), and about 80% brain-tissue water. The rigid skull allows very little space for expansion of these substances. When ICP increases to pathologic levels, brain damage can result.

The brain compensates for increases by regulating the three substances' volume by:

• limiting blood flow to the head
• displacing CSF into the spinal canal
• increasing absorption or decreasing production of CSF—pulling water out of brain tissue into the blood and excreting it through the kidneys. When compensatory mechanisms become overworked, small changes in volume lead to very large changes in pressure.

Here's a flow chart to help you understand increased ICP's pathophysiology.

Brain insult
• Trauma (contusion, laceration, intracranial hemorrhage), or
• Cerebral edema (following surgery, cerebrovascular accident, infection, hypoxia), or
• Hydrocephalus, or
• A space-occupying lesion (tumor, abscess)

↓

Slight increase in ICP

↓

Attempt at normal regulation of ICP by decreased blood flow to head

↓

Slight decrease in cerebral perfusion pressure (CPP)

↓

Loss of autoregulatory mechanism of constriction or dilation of cerebral blood vessels if increased ICP persists

↓

Passive dilation

Brain death

↑

Cellular hypoxia

↑

Uncal or central herniation | Further decrease in CPP

↑

Further increase in ICP

↑

Increased cerebral blood flow; venous congestion

NEUROLOGIC INJURIES

What to Do When Your Patient Has Increased Intracranial Pressure (ICP)

Your patient, Bill Curley, suffered a gunshot wound to his head. As you probably know, Mr. Curley needs treatment for increased ICP. The doctor will probably select one of the treatments below. Study this chart carefully to find out how each treatment works, and how you can help.

TREATMENT

ADMINISTRATION OF OSMOTIC DIURETICS, FOR EXAMPLE, MANNITOL (Osmitrol*) BY I.V. DRIP OR BOLUS

Purpose
• Reduces cerebral edema, decreasing intracranial contents
Nursing considerations
• Monitor fluids and electrolytes (including osmolarity) closely. Treatment may cause rapid dehydration.
• Watch for a rebound rise in ICP from treatment.
• Avoid storing mannitol at low temperatures, as it may crystallize.

ADMINISTRATION OF STEROIDS I.V.; FOR EXAMPLE, DEXAMETHASONE (Decadron*)

Purpose
• Reduces cerebral edema by lowering sodium and water concentration in the brain
Nursing considerations
• Give steroid with antacids orally and cimetidine (Tagamet*) orally or I.V., as ordered, to prevent peptic ulcers.
• Watch for signs and symptoms of gastrointestinal bleeding, such as dark-colored stools, low blood pressure, dizziness, nausea, and vomiting large amounts of bright red blood.

WITHDRAWAL OF CEREBRO-SPINAL FLUID (CSF) BY PERFORMING A LUMBAR OR CISTERNAL PUNCTURE, OR USING A VENTRICULAR CATHETER

Purpose
• Reduces CSF volume
Nursing considerations
• If the doctor performs a lumbar or cisternal puncture, perform a neurocheck frequently after the procedure. Remember, a sudden drop in ICP may allow brain herniation.
• If the doctor uses a ventricular catheter, prevent spesis by changing the tubing and drainage bag using strict aseptic technique.
Continued

*Available in both the U.S. and Canada

NEUROLOGIC INJURIES

What to Do When Your Patient Has Increased Intracranial Pressure (ICP)
Continued

RESTRICTION OF FLUID

Purpose
● Reduces cerebral edema and decreases brain volume, provided the brain's not diseased
Nursing considerations
● Monitor fluids and electrolytes (including osmolarity) closely. Dehydration below 325 Osm may have little therapeutic value.
● Maintain fluid restrictions according to the doctor's orders. (He'll probably restrict an adult patient to 1200 or 1500 ml/day.)
● Document the patient's fluid intake and output accurately. Remember to include all I.V. medications in your calculations.

HYPERVENTILATION WITH HAND-HELD RESUSCITATOR

Purpose
● Helps blow off CO_2 which causes constriction of blood vessels and reduction of cerebral blood flow
Nursing considerations
● Monitor arterial blood gas (ABG) measurement. Notify the doctor if CO_2 continues to rise. He may want to increase the rate of ventilations.

ADMINISTRATION OF BARBITURATES TO INDUCE COMA; FOR EXAMPLE, PHENOBARBITOL (Luminal*)

Purpose
● Decreases cerebral metabolic rate; decreases cerebral blood flow
Nursing considerations
● Monitor vital signs regularly, paying particular attention to respirations.
● Give barbiturates, as ordered. Remember, when performing neurochecks on your patient, you'll have difficulty assessing his mental status when he's receiving barbiturates.

SURGICAL REMOVAL OF SKULL BONE FLAP

Purpose
● Allows for expansion of cranial contents
Nursing considerations
● Keep the site of the surgical removal clean and dry to prevent infection.
● Maintain strict aseptic technique when redressing the site.

NEUROLOGIC INJURIES

Guide to Intracranial Pressure (ICP) Monitoring Systems

Does your patient need ICP monitoring? He may, if he has any of the following conditions:
• massive brain lesion
• head trauma with bleeding and edema
• overproduction and/or insufficient cerebrospinal fluid absorption, causing hydrocephalus
• congenital hydrocephalus
• cerebral hemorrhage
• encephalitis, particularly Reye's syndrome.

Also, suspect the need for ICP monitoring if you note signs of increased ICP pressure, such as with headache or vomiting, deteriorating respiratory pattern, deteriorating consciousness level, or deteriorating motor function.

Notify the doctor of any of these signs. He may decide to order ICP monitoring.

Monitoring systems

How familiar are you with ICP monitoring systems? For example, do you know the difference between a ventricular catheter and a subarachnoid screw?

This chart answers such questions and gives you specific information on the three most commonly used ICP monitoring devices. In addition, remember these general guidelines when setting up an ICP monitoring system:

Note: Procedures vary from hospital to hospital. Always follow your hospital's policy.
• Maintain strict aseptic technique throughout. Do everything possible to reduce the risk of infection.
• Keep all stopcock ports capped, unless you must open one to expel air or balance the transducer. Before you begin setting up, replace any open stopcock caps with closed ones.
• Expel air from the tubing and stopcock ports before connecting the line to the patient. Air in the line will damp the waveform, giving an inaccurate ICP reading.
• Never flush any fluid into the patient's cranial cavity. Doing so will raise his already elevated ICP and may also cause infection.

Continued

Guide to Intracranial Pressure (ICP) Monitoring Systems
Continued

VENTRICULAR CATHETER

Cannula and reservoir inserted into the brain's ventricle through a twist-drill hole in the skull.

Use
• To measure ICP
• To evaluate volume-pressure responses
• To drain large amount of cerebrospinal fluid (CSF)
• To instill contrast medium

Nursing considerations
• Expect catheter placement to be difficult if ventricle's collapsed, swollen, or displaced.
• Monitor patient closely for infections, such as meningitis and ventriculitis. Remember, this monitor is the most invasive of the three systems.
• Check catheter patency frequently. If catheter becomes occluded with blood or brain

tissue, notify the doctor. He may flush it with a small amount of sterile I.V. saline solution.
• Be sure stopcocks are positioned properly. Incorrect stopcock placement may create excessive CSF drainage, causing a sudden drop in ICP and possible brain herniation.
• Note any sudden changes in ICP reading. A collapsed ventricle may compress the catheter, causing a false reading.
• Recalibrate transducer and monitor frequently.

Advantages
• Direct CSF measurement
• Access for CSF drainage sampling
• Access for determining volume-pressure responses
• Access for antibiotic installation

Disadvantages
• Risk of infection
• Difficulty in locating the lateral ventricles in a patient with midline shifting or collapsed ventricles
• Risk of brain tissue damage

Continued

NEUROLOGIC INJURIES

Guide to Intracranial Pressure (ICP) Monitoring Systems
Continued

SUBARACHNOID SCREW

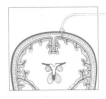

Steel screw with a sensor tip inserted through a twist-drill hole in skull. Small incision made in the dura mater allows screw and tip to connect with subarachnoid space. Transducer attached to screw converts CSF pressure to electrical impulses.

Use
• To measure ICP
• To provide access for CSF sampling

Nursing considerations
• Monitor patient closely for signs of infection.
• Recalibrate the transducer and monitor frequently.
• Check screw patency frequently. If screw becomes occluded with blood or brain tissue, notify the doctor. He may flush it with a small amount of sterile I.V. saline solution.

Advantages
• Direct measurement from CSF
• Access for CSF drainage or sampling
• Access for determining volume-pressure responses.

Disadvantages
• Risk of infection
• Requires skull firm enough to hold screw threads, as in patients over 6 years old
• Risk of screw plugging if skull swells.

Continued

NEUROLOGIC INJURIES

Guide to Intracranial Pressure (ICP) Monitoring Systems
Continued

EPIDURAL SENSOR

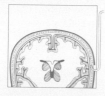

Tiny fiber-optic sensor inserted in brain's epidural space through burr hole in skull. Sensor cable plugs directly into monitor. Because this system cannot be recalibrated when affected by heat or pressure, its reliability remains controversial.

Use
• To measure ICP
Nursing considerations
• Monitor patient closely for infection. But remember, this monitor is the least invasive of the three systems.

• Check sensor's accuracy before each use. Set the monitor on "manual test" and apply a known pressure. If the readings aren't identical, discard the sensor. Obtain a new one and repeat the test.
• Be sure sensor's plugged tightly into monitor.
Advantages
• Less invasive.
Disadvantages
• Questionable reflection of CSF pressure
• No route for CSF drainage
• Volume-pressure responses not feasible.
Points to remember
• Irrigation is performed, when required, by the doctor.
• If you're assisting with irrigation, remember to use I.V. saline solution. *Never use the standard saline vials; they contain alcohol, which can cause cortical necrosis.*
• *Never use heparin:* The risk of small vessel bleeding is too great.

NEUROLOGIC INJURIES

Calibrating an ICP Monitor

To calibrate an intracranial pressure (ICP) monitor using the *cal factor*, first see if the cal factor is marked on the transducer. If not, obtain it by testing the transducer with a mercury sphygmomanometer, as the operator's manual directs. Depress the "balance" button. If the transducer is balanced properly, you'll get a zero reading. Release the button. Then, depress the "calibrate" button and, while holding this button down, use a screwdriver to turn the screw next to it until the digital reading equals the cal factor.

To use the *electric cal,* depress the "zero" button on the monitor. Make sure the

digital readout is zero and the oscilloscope line is at zero. Then depress the "test/cal" button and turn the "sensitivity" knob until the digital reading is 100 mm Hg and the line runs on the 100 mm Hg level.

To use the *pre-cal,* simply test the function of the monitor and transducer, because they're already calibrated with each other. Depress the "test" button and "zero" button simultaneously and hold them. The digital reading will be zero and the oscilloscope line will be at zero if the equipment's working properly.

Balance and calibrate the transducer and monitor at least once every 4 hours.

Complications

CNS infection, the most common hazard of ICP monitoring, can result from contamination of the equipment setup or of the insertion site.

Excessive loss of CSF can result from faulty stopcock placement or a drip chamber that's positioned too low.

Such loss can rapidly decompress the cranial contents and damage bridging cortical veins, leading to hematoma formation. Decompression can also lead to rupture of existing hematomas or aneurysms causing hemorrhage since it reduces the tamponade effect.

Applying a Head Bandage

1. Once the doctor has completed insertion of a cerebral catheter or subarachnoid screw for the purpose of intracranial pressure monitoring, he'll bandage the patient's head. You may be expected to change the dressing daily. Do you know how? If you're unsure, follow these guidelines.

Important: Be sure to maintain strict aseptic technique during the entire procedure.

2. Without handling the uncut gauze pads, saturate them with povidone-iodine solution. Now, remove the patient's old dressing and dispose of it properly, following your hospital's policy. Thoroughly wash your hands. After drying, put on your sterile gloves. Then, using the saturated pads, cleanse from the screw outward. As you're cleansing the area, examine the insertion site carefully for any signs of infection such as swelling, irritation, or drainage. If you note anything unusual, notify the doctor immediately following the dressing change.

3. Now, place the two precut drain sponges around the screw or catheter. Be sure that their edges overlap completely.

Note: Keep the screw or catheter exposed and easily accessible.

4. Next, secure the gauze pads with roller gauze. To do this, begin at the back of your patient's head, and wrap the stretch gauze bandage twice around his head. Then stop rolling the gauze when it's in the center of his forehead. Fold the gauze so it's pointing up, and begin laying it across the patient's crown.

5. Once you've reached the back of your patient's head, hold down the gauze with one finger. Then, reverse the procedure, bringing the gauze to the front of your patient's head. Repeat this process several times until one side of the head is covered by the gauze. Now, double the gauze back across the forehead to the other side.

6. Repeat the wrapping process on the other side of your patient's head, leaving the screw or catheter exposed and accessible.

7. Finally, wrap the roller gauze around your patient's head again, securing the folded corners. Secure the end of the gauze bandage with a single piece of adhesive tape. Wash your hands thoroughly. Document the dressing change and insertion site appearance in your nurses' notes.

Reading ICP Waveforms Accurately

1. *When you monitor a patient's intracranial pressure (ICP), you'll see some or all of the waveforms illustrated here.* Pictured first is a normal ICP waveform. Notice the steep upward systolic slope, followed by the downward diastolic slope with dicrotic notch. Ordinarily, this waveform occurs continuously and indicates an ICP measurement between 4 and 15 mm Hg.

2. The A waves shown here (sometimes called plateau waves) typically reach elevations of 50 to 100 mm Hg; and then drop sharply. They may come and go as the result of a temporary rise in thoracic pressure. But if they're recurring or are sustained for several minutes, A waves indicate a rapid, dangerous rise in ICP and a decreased ability to compensate. Consider such waves ominous. Notify the doctor at once. Sustained A waves may indicate irreversible brain damage.

3. The B waves illustrated here are sharp and rhythmic, with a sawtooth pattern. They occur every 1½ to 2 minutes and may reach elevations of 50 mm Hg. However, these high elevations aren't sustained. The clinical significance of B waves isn't clear,

Continued

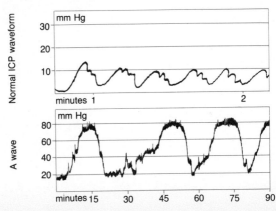

Reading ICP Waveforms Accurately
Continued

but they seem to occur more frequently with decreasing compensation. Sometimes, they precede A waves. Watch them closely, so you can notify the doctor promptly if such a change occurs.

4. C waves, as shown here, are rapid and rhythmic. They're less sharp in appearance than B waves, and may fluctuate with respirations or changing systemic blood pressure. C waves aren't clinically significant.

5. This illustration shows a damped waveform. This waveform tells you that the line's obstructed or that the transducer needs rebalancing. Locate the problem, and try to correct it.

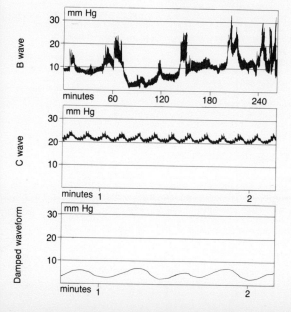

How to Troubleshoot a Damped Waveform

TRANSDUCER OR MONITOR NEEDS RECALIBRATION

Solution
• Turn stopcock off to patient.
• Open transducer's stopcock to air, and balance transducer.
• Recalibrate transducer and monitor.

AIR IN LINE

Solution
• Turn stopcock off to patient.
• Using a syringe, flush air out through an open stopcock port with sterile I.V. saline solution. *Note:* Never use heparin to flush the ICP line. You could accidentally inject some of the drug into the patient and cause bleeding.
• Rebalance and recalibrate transducer and monitor.

LOOSE CONNECTION IN LINE

Solution
• Check tubing and stopcocks for possible moisture, which may indicate a loose connection.
• Turn stopcock off to patient; then tighten all connections.
• Make sure the tubing's long enough to allow patient to turn his head without straining the tubing. This may prevent further problems.

DISCONNECTION IN LINE

Solution
• Turn stopcock off to patient *immediately*. (Rapid CSF loss through a ventricular catheter may allow ICP to drop precipitously, causing brain herniation.)
• Replace equipment to reduce risk of infection.

CHANGE IN PATIENT'S POSITION

Solution
• Reposition transducer's balancing port level with foramen of Monro.
• Rebalance and recalibrate transducer and monitor. *Remember:* Always balance and recalibrate at least once every 4 hours and whenever the patient's repositioned.

TUBING, CATHETER, OR SCREW OCCLUDED WITH BLOOD OR BRAIN TISSUE

Solution
• Notify doctor. He may want to irrigate the screw or catheter with a small amount (0.1 ml) of sterile I.V. saline solution. *Important:* Never irrigate the screw or catheter yourself.

Caring for the Patient on Intracranial Pressure (ICP) Monitoring

When you care for a critically ill patient, you probably try to schedule many nursing care procedures together. In this way, you avoid disturbing him repeatedly. But the patient suffering from high intracranial pressure (ICP) needs special consideration. Many nursing procedures—even routine ones, such as repositioning—tend to raise a patient's ICP. A cluster of nursing procedures done all at once may spike his ICP and produce menacing A waves. That's why you should do your best to schedule stressful procedures apart. Read this chart carefully. You'll see how certain stresses can endanger your patient. Then, you'll learn how to minimize them—or avoid them altogether.

MAINTAIN OXYGENATION; AVOID HYPOXIA AND/OR HYPERCAPNIA

Rationale
• A CO_2 excess and/or O_2 deficit in arterial blood stimulates cerebral vasodilation, increasing cerebral blood flow (CBF).
• Increasing CBF raises ICP.

Additional considerations
• Maintain a patent airway.
• Monitor arterial blood gas (ABG) measurements closely.
• If the doctor orders, hyperventilate the patient before suctioning, to minimize CO_2 accumulation during the procedure.
• Limit suctioning to 10 to 15 seconds.

MAINTAIN VENOUS OUTFLOW FROM THE BRAIN

Rationale
• Venous outflow increases capillary pressure and diminishes CSF absorption.
• Decreased outflow permits CO_2 and lactic acid to accumulate in the brain, stimulating cerebral vasodilation.
• ICP rises when venous outflow slows.
• As a response to rising ICP, blood pressure may drop, causing cerebral ischemia.

Additional considerations
• Do not place patient flat or in Trendelenburg position, unless the doctor orders. Instead, elevate the patient's head 30°, or as ordered.
• Keep the patient's head and neck midline to avoid compressing a jugular vein.

Continued

NEUROLOGIC INJURIES

Caring for the Patient on Intracranial Pressure (ICP) Monitoring
Continued

NEUROLOGIC INJURIES

MAINTAIN VENOUS OUT-
FLOW FROM THE BRAIN
Continued

• If the patient has an endotracheal tube in place, make sure
the tape securing it doesn't
compress the jugular veins.

PREVENT SYSTEMIC IN-
FECTION (sepsis)

Rationale
• Sepsis may produce in-
creased cardiac output and
vasodilation, increasing CBF.
Additional considerations
• Maintain scrupulous sterile
technique when doing daily
changes of equipment and
the patient's dressing.
• Get a CSF sample daily,
and send it for culturing. Before obtaining a sample from
the drainage bag, replace the
bag and tubing with sterile
ones. To prevent infection,
don't open the drainage bag
while it's attached to the patient.
• Notify doctor promptly if patient's temperature increases.

AVOID INCREASING INTRA-
THORACIC OR INTRA-
ABDOMINAL PRESSURE
(Valsalva maneuver)

Rationale
• Added thoracic or abdominal pressure can spike ICP
by increasing pressure on
central veins.
Additional considerations
• Don't put patient in Trendelenburg, unless ordered.
• Do not ask the patient to exe-
cute a Valsalva maneuver, even
during insertion of jugular or
subclavian vein catheter. Instead, expect the doctor to minimize the danger of air embolism
by using a syringe to apply suction to the catheter.
• Do your best to prevent the
patient from using the Valsalva
maneuver during bowel movements. Keep his stools soft with
an appropriate diet and/or stool
softeners. However, do not administer an enema.
• Prevent isometric muscular
contractions. Assist your patient when he sits up, and
instruct him not to push

Continued

Caring for the Patient on Intracranial Pressure (ICP) Monitoring
Continued

AVOID INCREASING INTRA-THORACIC OR INTRA-ABDOMINAL PRESSURE
Continued

against the bed's footboard. But if the doctor orders, encourage the patient to perform passive range-of-motion (ROM) excerises.
• Ask the patient to exhale when you turn him.
• Avoid hip flexion. When catheterizing a female patient, for example, flex her legs as little as possible.

PREVENT WIDE OR SUDDEN VARIATIONS IN SYSTEMIC BLOOD PRESSURE

Rationale
• Normally, autoregulation maintains cerebral perfusion pressure (CPP) at a level equal to mean systemic arterial pressure (MSAP) minus ICP. But autoregulation may fail when ICP is high. If so, CPP fluctuates with systemic blood pressure. Thus, an increase in systemic arterial

pressure (SAP) increases cerebral blood flow (CBF), elevates ICP, and worsens cerebral edema.
• Conversely, decreases in SAP may produce cerebral ischemia, allowing CO_2 and lactic acid to accumulate.
Additional considerations
• Use blood pressure and ICP monitors to evaluate the effect of stressful nursing procedures; for example, endotracheal tube insertion, suctioning, chest physiotherapy, and repositioning. Document your findings carefully.
• Minimize pain with a sedative or topical anesthetic, as ordered by the doctor.
• If ordered, use muscle relaxants to calm a combative patient during procedures like endotracheal tube insertion. However, avoid using restraints, unless ordered by the doctor.
• Rapid eye movement (REM) stages of sleep may cause a rise in ICP. Never perform stress-producing procedures during REM sleep.

NEUROLOGIC INJURIES

Causes of Hydrocephalus

Noncommunicating hydrocephalus. This hydrocephalus may result from *congenital* stenosis at the aqueduct of Sylvius, between the third and fourth ventricles; at the foramina of Luschka and/or Magendie, the outlets of the fourth ventricle (Dandy-Walker syndrome); or, rarely, at the foramina of Monro, passages of the lateral ventricles to the third ventricle.

Acquired stenosis of an aqueduct may result from fibrous adhesions, tumor, blood clot, or inflammatory scarring due to meningitis.

Communicating hydrocephalus. *Congenital* causes include leptomeningeal inflammation, which may lead to noncommunicating hydrocephalus if scar tissue forms an obstruction. Leptomeningeal inflammation may also be *acquired* from infection, hemorrhage, or particulate matter in CSF, all of which can occlude arachnoid villi, impairing CSF reabsorption.

Communicating hydrocephalus may also result from CSF overproduction. But since CSF can be reabsorbed much faster than it's formed, this cause is rare.

Normal-pressure hydrocephalus. Normal-pressure hydrocephalus is a type of communicating hydrocephalus most often seen in adults. In this hydrocephalus, ICP remains normal despite an increase in CSF that causes ventricular enlargement. Conditions that may lead to normal-pressure hydrocephalus include subarachnoid hemorrhage, arteriovenous malformation, or head trauma; thrombosis of the superior sagittal sinus; scarring of the basal cistern, usually secondary to head trauma or surgery; and bacterial meningitis.

Treating Hydrocephalus

Hydrocephalus is the cerebrospinal fluid (CSF) accumulation within the ventricular system, causing ventricular dilation. It stems from an imbalance between CSF production and reabsorption.

Although hydrocephalus may be acquired as a result of injury or disease, it's most often congenital. Congenital hydrocephalus, occurring in approximately 1 of every 1,000 births, may be nongenetic or genetic.

Continued

Treating Hydrocephalus
Continued

The most common surgical treatment for hydrocephalus is the ventriculoperitoneal shunt, although you may see a patient with a ventriculoatrial shunt. For the ventriculoperitoneal shunt, the doctor inserts a catheter into the patient's ventricular system, usually via a lateral ventricle. Then he attaches it to another catheter, which he tunnels through the subcutaneous tissue to a point below the diaphragm, where he can puncture the peritoneal sac. Between these catheters he places a valve system and inserts it under the patient's scalp, behind his ear.

Preoperative and postoperative care of a shunt patient is the same as for a craniotomy patient.

After the shunt's in place, an infant may be irritable. An older child may get headaches when he tries to sit up. Help him to sit up by gradually raising his head in stages, about 20° at a time. Reassure him that his headaches will stop when he's accustomed to the shunt.

Before discharge, give the patient's family clear instructions about his shunt. Tell them to report at once any symptoms of increased ICP, such as restlessness, headaches, or decreased level of consciousness. These may indicate that the shunt is blocked.

They should also call the doctor immediately if signs of infection occur: increased temperature, headaches, or nuchal rigidity.

Regardless of the cause, the prognosis in hydrocephalus is poor if the condition remains untreated. Without surgery, hydrocephalus leads to increased intracranial pressure (ICP), which is potentially fatal; in infants, the associated infection and malnutrition can also have serious consequences. In all patients, the prognosis depends on the underlying cause, its severity, and the effectiveness of treatment.

Continued

NEUROLOGIC INJURIES

Treating Hydrocephalus
Continued

VENTRICULOPERITONEAL SHUNT

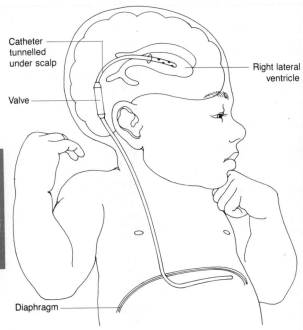

Catheter
tunnelled
under scalp

Valve

Right lateral
ventricle

Diaphragm

What Happens in Coma

Coma isn't just unconsciousness, but unconsciousness from which the patient can't be aroused by even strong stimulation. The brain's reticular activating system (RAS)—an intricate network of connections extending from a brain stem center to the hypothalamus, thalamus, and cerebral cortex—is disturbed, preventing the intercommunication that makes consciousness and active motor function possible. Because the RAS is centered in the brain stem core and fans out over the cortex, insult or injury to different areas of the brain affects consciousness in different ways.

Consciousness is altered by two pathologic mechanisms broadly classified as those that widely depress cerebral hemisphere function and those that specifically depress or destroy areas of the brain stem RAS. For example, significant bilateral cerebral hemisphere damage may produce the same effect on consciousness as a pinhead-sized brain stem injury.

Coma-producing processes are further classified by the regions they affect:
• *Supratentorial*—for example, intracerebral, epidural, or subdural hematoma; arterial (thrombotic or embolic), or venous occlusions; tumors; abscesses
• *Subtentorial*—for example, cerebellar hemorrhage, infarct, or abscess; brain stem infarct or aneurysm; pons hemorrhage
• *Metabolic or diffuse brain dysfunction*—for example, anoxia, hypoglycemia, uremia, electrolyte imbalance, liver failure, or endocrine disorders; drug toxicity; cardiogenic or hypovolemic shock.

Some severe psychiatric disorders can also produce a coma-like state (psychogenic unresponsiveness).

NEUROLOGIC INJURIES

Special Consideration

Just because your patient's comatose doesn't mean he can't hear. Remember to:
Treat him with dignity.
• Don't discuss his condition when standing by his bedside.
• Don't perform a procedure without telling him first.
Keep him stimulated.
• Talk to him, and encourage his family and other staff members to do so.
• Suggest to his family that they tapercord messages at home and play them at his bedside.

Common Causes Of Coma

CHEMICAL
Alcohol
Carbon dioxide and carbon monoxide narcosis
Anoxia
TRAUMATIC
Skull fracture
Subdural hematoma
Subarachnoid hemorrhage
Brain stem injury
INFECTIOUS
Syphilis of the CNS
Meningitis—viral or bacterial
Encephalitis
VASCULAR
Cerebral aneurysm (berry) and/or
rupture
Cerebral tumor
Cerebral vascular lesions
Cardiac decompensation
Shock—hemorrhagic, septic, hypovolemic
OTHER
Diabetes
Hepatic failure
Electrolyte disorders
Deficiencies of thiamine and vitamin B_{12}
Poisoning
Seizures
Uremia

Priorities for Treating Coma

Your first nursing priority is to ensure adequate perfusion and oxygenation of the patient's brain and other vital organs. You can do this while you perform a thorough assessment and evaluate the results of his laboratory studies.

Although the patient's airway and respirations were stabilized initially, remember that his respiratory status can deteriorate suddenly at any time while he's unconscious. If his respiratory status worsens, and if he was given oxygen earlier, he may need to be given a higher percentage of oxygen now. Or, if he wasn't intubated and placed on a

ventilator earlier, this may have to be done now. Observe your patient carefully, and always keep airways and intubation equipment on hand. To prevent aspiration of vomitus, a nasogastric tube will be inserted.

Continue to check your comatose patient for signs and symptoms of internal or external bleeding. A central venous pressure line may be inserted for accurate evaluation of the patient's hemodynamic status and for fluid infusion. You'll insert an indwelling (Foley) catheter to help you evaluate his output.

NEUROLOGIC INJURIES

Spinal Cord Trauma

SPINAL CORD INJURY (contusion, compression, complete transection of cord)

CHIEF COMPLAINT

• *Motor disturbances:* with contusion and compression, muscle weakness or paralysis; with complete transection, permanent motor paralysis below level of lesion; with upper motor neuron damage, spastic paralysis; with lower motor neuron damage, flaccid paralysis
• *Sensory deviations:* related to size of injury and degree of cord shock; absence of perspiration on affected part; with contusion or compression, pain at level of lesion; with complete transection, total sensory loss

HISTORY

• Auto and motorcycle accidents, athletic injuries (football, diving), falls, gunshot wounds, stab wounds
• Cervical injuries most common

PHYSICAL EXAMINATION

• Urinary retention, priapism, perspiration on one side; first 24 to 48 hours, flaccid paralysis, then exaggerated reflexes or spastic paralysis if lower motor neuron remains intact
• Specific levels of injury intact and functional loss: with C1 to C2, quadriplegic, no respiratory ability; C3 to C4, quadriplegic, loss of phrenic innervation to diaphragm, absent respirations; C4 to C5, quadriplegic, no arm movements; C5 to C6, quadriplegic, gross arm movements only; C6 to C7, quadriplegic, biceps movement, no triceps movement; C7 to C8, quadriplegic, triceps, no intrinsic muscles of hands; thoracic L1 to L2, arm function intact, loss of some intercostals, and loss of leg, bladder, bowel, sex function; lumbar below L2, motor and sensory loss, impairment of bladder, bowel, sex function according to nerve root damage; sacral, loss of bladder, bowel, sex function

NEUROLOGIC INJURIES

Special Consideration

If your patient's cord injury is between *C1 and C4*, he'll be completely unable to breathe; ventilate him with an Ambu bag until he can be intubated and mechanically ventilated. Usually, a doctor highly skilled in intubation will perform the procedure. The patient with this type of cord injury will require lifelong ventilation and supportive care.

If the patient's injury is in the *C4 to C8* area, he'll be breathing diaphragmatically and probably won't need immediate intubation.

Spinal Cord Emergencies

RUPTURED INTRAVERTEBRAL DISC

Cause
● Trauma
Signs and symptoms
● When trauma occurs in lumbar area, patient has pain in lower back, radiating down back of one leg. Also patient's paravertebral muscles are spastic, and his affected leg can't be straightened when his thigh is flexed.
● When trauma occurs in cervical area, patient has neck stiffness and local pain radiating down one arm to fingers.
Emergency nursing considerations
● Place patient in pelvic or cervical traction, if ordered.

● Prepare patient for myelogram, as ordered.
● Prepare patient for a laminectomy, if ordered.
● Give pain medication, as ordered.
HYPEREXTENSION INJURY
Falls causing backward thrust of the head or rear-end automobile collisions causing acceleration injuries in which sudden, forceful impact and forward movement hyperextend the neck
PENETRATING INJURY
Bullet, stab, or other penetrating wound that causes damage to spinal cord tissue and blood vessels

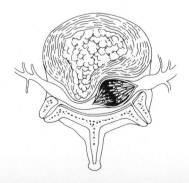

Spinal Cord Lesions

TRAUMATIC LESIONS

Burst injury
Automobile accident or any direct force which is great enough to shatter the vertebral body, causing bone chips to injure the cord.

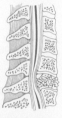

Flexion injury
Anterior
Automobile accidents, generally head-on collisions; falls in which the back of the head receives the force of impact, causing hyperflexion of the neck.

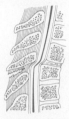

Compression injury
Accidents from diving, surfing, or trampolining, causing vertical blow to head. Resulting dislocation injures the cord.

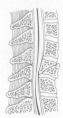

Flexion-rotation injury
Automobile accidents, falls, or accidents during contact sports or skiing that cause deformation injuries in which spinal cord-supporting structures cannot accommodate movement

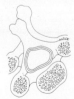

Understanding Spinal Cord Syndromes

If the spinal cord is partially severed, clinical picture may reflect all or some of the signs and symptoms of one or several of the syndromes shown below.

CENTRAL CORD SYNDROME
● Results from hyperextension or flexion injuries
● Causes greater loss of motor function in the patient's arms than in his legs
● Causes slight sensory loss

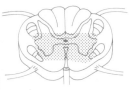

BROWN-SÉQUARD SYNDROME
● Results from flexion-rotation injuries or from penetration injuries
● Causes complete motor loss on the ipsilateral side of the patient's injury
● Causes complete loss of pain and temperature sensation on the contralateral side of injury

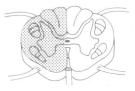

ANTERIOR CORD SYNDROME
● Usually results from flexion injuries
● Causes loss of upper and lower motor neuron function (voluntary and reflex motor activity)
● Causes loss of temperature and pain sensation
● Causes *no* loss of patient's ability to sense light touch, vibration, and pressure

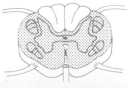

POSTERIOR CORD SYNDROME
● Results from cervical hyperextension injuries
● Causes loss of light touch sensation and proprioception
● Motor function of extremities preserved

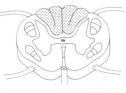

Assessing Level of a Spinal Cord Lesion

ASK THE PATIENT TO...	OBSERVE AND TEST BODY PART	LEVEL ASSOCIATED WITH MOTION	LEVEL ASSOCIATED WITH SENSATION
Shrug his shoulders; take a deep breath	Shoulder, chest, and abdomen	C3 to C5	C4
Bend his elbow	Elbow	C5	Radial side C6 Ulnar side T1
Bend his wrist up	Wrist	C6	C6 (thumb side of wrist)
Oppose his thumb to each fingertip; make a fist	Thumb First two digits Little finger	C8 to T1	C6 C7 T1
Tighten his abdomen	Abdomen Pubis Navel Nipple line	T5 to T12	L1 T10 T4
Flex his hip	Hips	L1 to L3	L2
Straighten his leg	Knees	L2 to L4	L3
Bend and straighten his toes	Toes	L5, S1, and S2	L5
Tighten his sphincter muscle around your finger	Perineum	S2 to S4	S5

NEUROLOGIC INJURIES

Functional Goals in Spinal Cord Lesions

SPINAL CORD LEVEL	MUSCLE FUNCTION	FUNCTIONAL GOALS
C3—4	Neck control; scapular elevators	• Manipulate electric wheelchair with mouth stick. • Limited self-feeding with ballbearing feeders.
C5	Fair to good shoulder control; good elbow flexion	• Dress upper trunk. • Turn bed with arm slings. • Propel manual wheelchair with hand-rim projections or electric wheelchair with hand controls. • Self-feeding with hand splints. • Assist getting to and from bed.
C6	Good shoulder control; wrist extension; supinators	• Transfer from wheelchair to bed and auto with or without minimal assistance. • Self-feeding with tenodesis hands • Assist getting to and from commode chair.
C7	Weak shoulder depression; weak elbow extension; some hand function	• Independent in transfer to bed, car, and toilet. • Total dressing independence. • Wheelchair without hand-rim projections. • Self-feeding.
C8 to T4	Good to normal upper extremity muscle function	• Wheelchair to floor and return. • Wheelchair up and down curb. • Wheelchair to tub and return.
T5 to L2	Partial to good trunk stability	• Total wheelchair independence. • Limited ambulation with bilateral long-leg braces and crutches.

Continued

NEUROLOGIC INJURIES

Functional Goals in Spinal Cord Lesions
Continued

SPINAL CORD LEVEL	MUSCLE FUNCTION	FUNCTIONAL GOALS
L3 to L4	All trunk-pelvic stabilizers intact; hip flexors; adductors; quadriceps	• Ambulation with short-leg braces with or without crutches, depending on level.
L5 to S3	Hip extensors; abductors; knee flexors; ankle control	• No equipment needed if plantar flexion enough for push off at end of stance.

How to Manage Autonomic Dysreflexia (AD)

You'll want to be able to understand and recognize AD (hyperreflexia), so you'll be better prepared to care for your patient. Why? Without prompt action to remove the stimulus and decrease the patient's blood pressure, AD may cause seizures, intracranial hemorrhage, and even death.

What causes AD? This complication develops in about 85% of patients with spinal cord lesions at the T_6 level or above. The three most common stimuli include:
• Bladder stimulation from overdistention, either caused by a kinked or blocked catheter, an improperly positioned drainage bag, or urine back-up. Bladder spasms or stones, urinary tract infection, or manual stimu-

lation procedures, such as catheterization and irrigation, may also stimulate the bladder.
• Bowel stimulation from overdistention caused by a fecal impaction, constipation, or excess gas. Other possible stimuli are a rectal exam, manual evacuation, an enema, or suppository insertion.
• Skin stimulation caused by improper turning and position, or from treatment manipulation. Autonomic dysreflexia may also be triggered by extreme cold or heat; pressure on the glans penis or testicles; decubitus ulcers; or an ingrown toenail.

Keep in mind that AD may de-

Continued

NEUROLOGIC INJURIES

How to Manage Autonomic Dysreflexia (AD)
Continued

velop suddenly anytime after a spinal injury. Physical reaction to AD is immediate. Its signs and symptoms include: extreme blood pressure elevation; sweating and flushing above the lesion level; chills, gooseflesh, and pale skin below the lesion level; nasal stuffiness; nausea; severe headache; blurred vision; rapid pulse rate which then slows; and metallic taste.

How can AD be managed before it seriously affects your patient? Consider it critical to immediately lower his blood pressure. To do so, elevate the head of his bed to a 45° angle, or help him into a sitting position, unless contraindicated.

Note: Placing a quadriplegic in a sitting position automatically decreases his blood pressure.

Then notify the doctor. Monitor his blood pressure every 3 to 5 minutes and take immediate action to eliminate the stimulus.

Check to make sure your patient isn't sitting or lying on his catheter, tubing, or drainage bag. Then, check for any obstruction. Palpate his bladder for overdistention. Is his bladder distended? If so, and your patient doesn't have a catheter and can't urinate, gently catheterize him.

Caution: To prevent additional

abdominal pressure, never use Credé's maneuver.

If his urine flow is intact and the symptoms persist, check for bowel stimulation. Is your patient impacted? Gently remove the impaction, then apply dibucaine hydrochloride ointment (Nupercainal Ointment*) or lidocaine hydrochloride jelly (Xylocaine Jelly) to his rectum after all the symptoms subside. If he's not impacted, ask him some questions. When was his last bowel movement? Was it hard or soft? Has he had a recent enema? Had a suppository inserted?

If his bladder and bowel are not the sources of the stimulation, check for skin stimulation. Is a sharp object irritating your patient's skin? Have pressure areas developed from leaving him in one position too long? If so, remove the source of pressure or stimulation.

Suppose the symptoms continue to persist 1 to 2 minutes after you've removed the stimulus. Then, you may be ordered by the doctor to administer medications I.V., such as phentolamine methanesulfonate (Regitine), hydralazine hydrochloride (Apresoline*), or diazoxide (Hyperstat*). Continue to monitor your patient's

*Available in both the U.S. and Canada.

Continued

How to Manage Autonomic Dysreflexia (AD)
Continued

blood pressure 3 to 4 hours after the symptoms subside. Remember, his blood pressure may drop rapidly or AD may recur.

After your patient's condition has stabilized, teach him how to recognize the signs and symptoms of AD. Advise him to contact a doctor immediately if he feels any of AD's warning signals. Explain to him the importance of a planned bladder and bowel program, and the need for proper body turning and positioning. Remind your patient to periodically check his catheter, tubing, and bag for possible blockage or kinked tubing.

Spinal Surgery

LAMINECTOMY
In this procedure, the surgeon makes an incision over the involved vertebral area and extends it down through fascia and muscles to the laminae (flattened parts on sides of vertebral arch). Then he removes one or more laminae or portions of them.

Surgeons perform a laminectomy to reach dura, disc, or cord, and complete needed surgery in those areas.
Postoperative nursing care:
• Your patient may get out of bed within 24 hours after surgery, although this isn't always so.
• Check for: hemorrhage; motor or sensory deficits; loss of bowel or bladder functioning.
• Position as ordered; maintain alignment; log-roll when turning.
SPINAL FUSION
Occasionally, after laminectomy, the patient needs spinal fusion.

For example, this may be needed if a lesion or injury has caused an unstable spine. To accomplish spinal fusion, the surgeon will remove bone from part of the patient's body (usually the iliac crest) and graft it onto the vertebrae.
Postoperative nursing care:
• Prepare patient for possible extended bedrest in flat position. Tell him he'll have to wear a back brace when he gets out of bed.
• Prevent movement at fusion site. Position the patient as ordered, maintain alignment, and log-roll when turning.
• Check for hemorrhage; motor or sensory deficits; and loss of bowel or bladder functioning. Occasionally, a surgeon inserts Harrington rods after spinal fusion. These act as temporary internal splints to help the bones unite properly.

NEUROLOGIC INJURIES

Sexuality and Spinal Cord Injury

When a person becomes paralyzed, his sexual apprehensions are likely to start right away, not weeks or months after he's been transferred to a rehabilitation center. Because his feelings of self-worth and accomplishment are so closely tied to self-image and sexuality, anything that alters that image will mar his sense of personal fulfillment. Unless you acknowledge your patient's sexual anxiety quickly and attempt to deal with it, he may lose interest in all rehabilitation therapy. That's why your role in counseling's so important.

Obviously, you're not a psychologist. Nevertheless, you can talk to your patient as one human being to another and help him communicate his fears and hopes. Of course, to do this, you must first have come to terms with sexuality yourself. Answer all questions truthfully and calmly. If your patient confronts you with a question you can't answer, say you don't know but you'll find out.

To help your patient understand how his spinal injury will affect him sexually, be prepared to explain how his nervous system's been damaged and what level of sexual functioning he can expect. If you know the kind and extent of his injury, you can estimate how much physiological sexual capability remains. For example, in complete cord injuries, loss of genital sensation occurs, although this doesn't necessarily mean loss of sexual pleasure. Most males with upper motor neuron injuries can have reflexogenic erections with cutaneous stimulation. Males with lower motor neuron injuries, however, will not have reflexogenic erections but may have psychogenic erections through erotic stimulation via sight, sound, smell, and touch. Male fertility is drastically reduced, since the nervous synchronization needed for ejaculation is disrupted.

Females with upper motor neuron lesions will have reflex clitoral engorgement and vaginal lubrication with local stimulation. Females with lower motor neuron lesions may need to use external lubrication.

Female fertility remains unchanged: A woman with spinal cord injuries can have normal pregnancies with vaginal deliveries. But a woman with an upper motor neuron disorder may experience dysreflexia during labor.

Both patient and partner will face difficult adjustments and may benefit from continued professional counseling. Whatever activity the couple engages in must meet the approval of both partners. They must feel that sex is natural and normal: an expression of themselves and their desire to share intimacy.

Learning about Sexual Options

To help your patient with a neurologic disorder thoroughly enjoy sexual experiences, you'll need to make him aware of sexual possibilities.

Here are some points to review with your patient:
• If your patient has functional use of his hands, tell him he can use his hands to sexually stimulate, or even satisfy his partner.
• If your patient doesn't have functional use of his hands, suggest oral sexual options involving sucking, nibbling, and tongue stimulation of each other's bodies.
• Because of your patient's physical limitations, recommend experimenting with sexual positions.
• If your patient has a catheter, remind him that it's not always necessary to remove it before intercourse. After the penis is erect, the catheter may be bent and folded along the penile shaft. If your patient's female, the catheter can be pushed aside and positioned out of the way.
• If your patient has an ostomy, recommend he empty the pouch before sexual intercourse. Your patient may also want to use a pouch cover.
• If your patient's female, and has vaginal lubrication difficulties, suggest she use a water-soluble lubricant, such as K-Y Brand Lubricating Jelly.
• To get better motion during sexual activity, recommend the patient and partner consider a water bed. Another way to achieve better movement is to take advantage of muscle spasms.

If your patient has paraplegia, quadraplegia, or can't always maintain an erection, familiarize him with the following mechanical aids. *The penis stiffener* is usually made of a formed piece of hard rubber that fits over the patient's penis and holds it erect. *The dildo* is an artificial penis, usually made of semihard rubber, that is strapped on or above the penis. A dildo can also be hand-held. *The vibrator* is an artificial penis made of hard plastic. It is battery-operated and is hand-held. *The flexible rubber sheath* can be placed over the vibrator for greater vaginal or anal stimulation.

NEUROLOGIC INJURIES

Using Traction (Skull Tongs or Halo Vest) to Immobilize a Spinal Cord-Injured Patient

SKULL TONGS

Used to immobilize the patient's cervical spine after fracture or dislocation, invasion by tumor or infection, or surgery

Nursing considerations
• Reassure the patient and explain the procedure to him.
• Assess his neurologic signs, as ordered, with particular emphasis on motor function. Notify the doctor *immediately* if the patient experiences decreased sensation or increased loss of motor function: this may indicate *spinal cord trauma*.
• Be alert for signs and symptoms of loosening pins: redness, swelling, and complaints of persistent pain and tenderness. (Causes of loosening pins include infection, excessive traction force, and osteoporosis.)
• If the pins pull out, immobilize the patient's head and neck and call the doctor.
• Take action to prevent pressure sores. Remember, inadequate peripheral circulation can cause sores within 6 hours.
• Make sure the traction weights are hanging freely to maintain proper traction force. *Never add or subtract weights unless the doctor orders it.* (Inappropriate weight adjustment may cause neurologic impairment.)

HALO-VEST TRACTION

Used to immobilize the patient's head and neck after cervical spine injury (allows greater mobility than skull tongs; carries less risk of infection)

Nursing considerations
• Reassure the patient and explain the procedure to him.
• Assess his neurologic signs, as ordered, with particular emphasis on motor function. Notify the doctor *immediately* if the patient experiences decreased sensation or increased loss of motor function: this may indicate *spinal cord trauma*.
• Check the pin sites and use cleansing procedures, as ordered.
• Obtain an order for an analgesic if your patient complains of headache after the doctor retightens the pins.
• Never lift the patient using the device's bars.

Caring for a Patient in Cervical Traction

Cervical traction is applied following fractures or dislocations of the cervical or high thoracic vertebrae. Tongs attached to the patient's skull are used with a weight-and-pulley system to exert pull along the axis of the spine. This arrangement promotes vertebral alignment and decreases the possibility of inadvertent movement and further injury. However, it does carry the risk of spinal cord injury from excessive manipulation of the patient's head and cervical vertebrae during traction application.

Three types of tongs are used in cervical spine traction: Gardner-Wells, Crutchfield, and Vinke. Gardner-Wells tongs are considered the least likely of the three to slip and tear the skin from prolonged use, or use with excessive amounts of weight.

If you're caring for a patient in cervical traction, provide the following special care:
• Turn your patient as soon as possible after the skull tongs are applied and the desired vertebral alignment has been confirmed by an X-ray. Use a special bed or frame, such as the Circle® bed or Stryker frame, so you can turn your patient without disrupting vertebral alignment.
• Monitor your patient's blood pressure, pulse, respiratory rate, and temperature every hour until stable, and then every 2 to 4 hours thereafter. Remember, low systolic blood pressure (90 mmHg and below) is one indication of spinal cord trauma. Also, respiratory complications are more common with high cervical injury.

Continued

NEUROLOGIC INJURIES

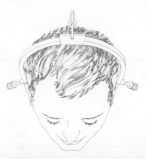

Caring for a Patient in Cervical Traction
Continued

• Note the degree and location of pain, paresthesia, paralysis, or loss of muscle power, before tong application, and hourly for the first 24 hours following tong application. Continue assessment thereafter according to doctor's orders.

• Check the tongs often for correct placement.

• Perform pin care at the tong insertion sites, depending on hospital policy or doctor's orders. Expect only minimal bleeding at these sites following application, since the anesthetic of choice contains epinephrine. Notify the doctor if bleeding persists.

• Observe and frequently assess all bony prominences, including the heels, elbows, and occipital area.

• Provide meticulous skin care and position changes every 2 hours, unless contraindicated, especially if your patient has any sensory or motor function loss.

• If ordered by the doctor, provide padding or support under your patient's head, neck, or shoulders.

• Encourage your patient to feed himself, if possible. Turn him on his side for feeding. Supply a high-protein and high-caloric diet, or a soft diet if it's painful for your patient to chew.

• Provide rectal stimulation, as ordered, for bowel function.

• Provide emotional and moral support for your patient and his family. They'll probably be particularly anxious, considering the implications of spinal cord injury.

• Document all your care in your nurses' notes.

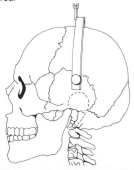

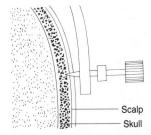

Scalp

Skull

Safe Transport

Moving an accident victim with possible spinal cord injury can be hazardous unless his head, neck, and thoracic spine are kept aligned. By providing constant cervical spine traction, the Meyer cervical orthosis allows healthcare professionals to resuscitate, turn, and transport such a patient with less risk of further injury.

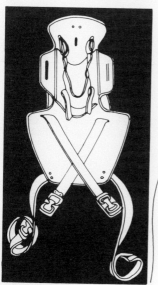
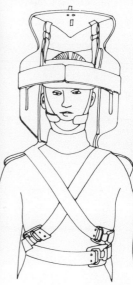

Turning Your Patient on Stryker Frames and Beds

Frames and beds
To care for a patient with spinal cord injuries who's immobilized on a frame or bed, you'll need to know the following: how to maintain proper spinal alignment; how to prevent further spinal cord damage; and how to promote healing of his bony injury. Additionally, you must take measures to prevent skin breakdown and contracture deformities.

NEUROLOGIC INJURIES

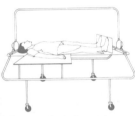

1 Proper patient alignment
supine position

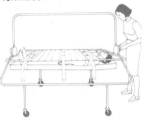

2 Frame secured with safety straps over patient

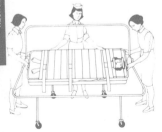

3 Turning the patient

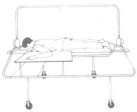

4 Turn accomplished. Proper patient alignment
prone position

Continued

Turning Your Patient on Stryker Frames and Beds
Continued

Stryker frame—A patient with severe neck or back injuries may be immobilized on a Stryker frame. Make sure you explain the purpose of the frame to your patient and his family; it will probably seem frightening to them. Unless your patient's prepared, he may fear falling when he's turned.

The Stryker frame uses an anterior and a posterior frame with canvas covers and thin padding over each. The frames, which are supported on a movable cart, have a pivot apparatus at each end. This allows you to change the patient's position to either prone or supine without altering his alignment.

To do this properly, follow the manufacturer's instructions or your hospital's procedure manual.

Further tips: Before turning your patient, secure any equipment he may have, such as I.V.s, Foley catheter, or respirator tubing to make sure it'll easily turn with him.

Some patients prefer to be turned more quickly than others. Place your patient's preference on his care plan along with the turning schedule.

• To prevent malalignment, check the equipment periodically and tighten the lacing of the canvases.

• To protect your patient's skin, place a foam mattress or padding on both frames and cover it with sheepskin.

• To aid in maintaining proper alignment, use a footboard, hand roll, bolsters and splints, as required.

• You may add arm rest wings to the frame at shoulder level. They'll permit your patient to rest his arms and will help maintain alignment.

• For meals, place him in prone position.

• For elimination, place him in supine position, with his bedpan under the opening in the canvas.

• When your patient's prone, carefully watch him for signs of respiratory problems. This position makes breathing more difficult.

Continued

NEUROLOGIC INJURIES

Turning Your Patient on Stryker Frames and Beds
Continued

• Help prevent your patient from feeling isolated, especially when he's prone. If he likes TV, place a set on the floor. Can he move his arms? He may wish to have books or hobbies on a tray under the frame.

• To care for a patient with skull tongs on a Stryker frame, always maintain traction, even when turning. During the turn, the nurse positioned at the patient's head will check pulley and weights.

Circle bed—You may be caring for a patient with neck or back injuries who's immobilized in a Circle bed. This is a revolving bed with two major parts: a bottom mattress and a turning stretcher. A large, circular metal frame surrounds your patient, letting you turn him as often as necessary with minimal trauma or extraneous movement. To operate the bed electrically, you simply depress a push button. However, you can also operate it manually, if necessary.

As you can see in the photo above, your patient lies "sandwiched" between the bottom mattress and the turning stretcher, which you have secured over him.

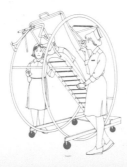

Continued

NEUROLOGIC INJURIES

Turning Your Patient on Stryker Frames and Beds
Continued

You change his position by turning him through an arc of the circle. *To minimize nausea and vertigo, don't interrupt the turn until he reaches the desired position.* For specific instructions on the turning procedure, consult the manufacturer's instructions or your hospital's procedure manual. *Nursing tips:*

• Familiarize patient and family with the Circle bed so they won't be frightened by it.

• Before turning your patient, make sure I.V. lines and other equipment aren't tangled.

• Have another nurse help you turn your patient. One of you should operate the push button while the other watches the patient.

• If your patient has skull tongs, maintain traction during the turn. Make sure the equipment's secured to the mobile portion of the frame so it moves easily with him. Watch that the pulley clears the frame during the turn.

• For elimination, secure a bedpan to an opening on mattress or frame, depending on your patient's position.

• If the patient has copious respiratory drainage, provide a basin to collect secretions.

• When the patient's supine, give him prism glasses to increase his field of vision. With these, he can see all activity at eye level. If he can move his arms, he'll be able to read by holding a book normally, rather than overhead.

• To increase your patient's field of vision, attach a mirror to the upper part of the bed. Remember to remove it before turning him.

• In the prone position, a patient who has arm movement can take care of oral hygiene, write letters, play a game of solitaire, or read. Place the necessary materials on an overbed table within his reach.

Roto Rest bed—Suppose you're caring for a patient who's immobilized on a Roto Rest bed. Equipped with supportive packs and straps that keep the patient's body in proper alignment, this bed gently and continually rocks

Continued

Turning Your Patient on Stryker Frames and Beds
Continued

him in a cradle-like fashion. Besides alleviating the need for turning and positioning, the bed reduces risk of fecal impaction and constipation. Consult manufacturer's instructions and hospital procedure manual for guidelines.

Nursing tips: After bathing patient, make sure soap residue's rinsed off his body and support pack.

• Before turning patient, replace all packs and secure straps.

• For elimination, place bedpan under opening in bed.

• Bed's continuous motion promotes postural drainage, so be prepared to suction patient frequently during his first 48 hours on bed.

Clinitron bed—You may care for a patient who's immobilized on an air-fluidized support system. A rectangular frame containing silicone-coated glass beads (microspheres) covered with a monofilament polyester sheet makes up this special bed. Warm pressurized air fluidizes beads. This bed provides a clean, controlled environment and reduces contact pressure.

Refer to manufacturer's instructions and hospital procedure when caring for patient on this bed. Also read these guidelines:

• If a dressing's necessary, keep it as small as possible.

• If patient has excessive wound drainage, place porous dressing under wound.

• Clean system every week.

• For elimination, roll patient away from you and push bedpan into microspheres. Reposition patient on bedpan. Afterward, defluidize system and remove bedpan by holding it flat as you roll patient away from you with your other hand. Cleanse patient, as usual. Fluidize system and reposition patient.

Regular hospital bed—For position changes, one person stands at head of bed to guide patient's head and traction pulley. Two other people move patient with pull sheet to one side of bed, then carefully log-roll him onto side. To prevent lateral flexion, place small foam block under patient's head while he's on his side.

Dealing with Daily-Care Complications

Immobility poses special complication risks. Since the patient with a neurologic injury is usually immobilized or on bed rest, you must be particularly alert for these complications. This chart lists some of the complications by body system of immobility that your patient may experience. It also details the action you can take to prevent or minimize these problems. Don't forget: If you must perform any of these intervention procedures, be sure you explain to the patient beforehand what you're going to do and why.

NEUROLOGIC SYSTEM

Complications
• Dependency
• Disorientation
• Decreased motivation
• Insomnia
• Decreased learning
• Decreased memory
• Apathy
• Withdrawal
• Frustration
• Anger
• Aggression
• Regression

Nursing interventions
• Gradually increase your patient's physical activities. Encourage independency by allowing him to co-manage his care and do as much for himself as possible. Keep him involved and informed on all aspects of his care and therapy
• Hold frequent conversations with your patient to maintain orientation. Have clocks and calendars in his room. Turn lights off at night.

• Provide your patient with intellectual stimulation. For example, encourage his family to visit, and suggest he read newspapers, books, and magazines, or work crossword puzzles.
• Discourage your patient from taking excessively frequent daytime naps.
• Provide sensory stimulation, such as familiar pictures, ceiling posters, music, or talking books.
• Encourage physical and occupational therapy, as indicated.
• Provide privacy when performing any procedures.
• Spend time with your patient; answer all questions.

INTEGUMENTARY SYSTEM(skin)

Complications
• Painful, reddened areas
• Decubitus ulcers
• Infection

Nursing interventions
• Turn and position your patient regularly, if patient can't do it himself.

Continued

NEUROLOGIC INJURIES

Dealing with Daily-Care Complications
Continued

NEUROLOGIC INJURIES

INTEGUMENTARY SYSTEM
Continued

• Make sure your patient is on a high-protein, low-calcium diet, with plenty of fluids.
• Observe all skin surfaces, especially bony prominences, for pressure signs, such as blanched or reddened areas. Gently massage reddened areas (especially over bony prominences) to stimulate circulation.
• Keep your patient's skin clean and dry.
• Whenever possible, use a draw-sheet or sheepskin to move your patient to avoid irritating his skin.
• When necessary, use special equipment to minimize pressure on your patient's body: an egg crate, air, or water mattress; flotation pads; or heel and elbow protectors.
• Use positioning aids, as needed.
• If the patient does develop a decubitus ulcer, care for it frequently, as ordered.
• If patient has a decubitus ulcer, watch him closely for signs of septicemia, such as increased temperature and purulent drainage. Take cultures, as indicated.
• Administer antibiotics, as ordered.

MUSCULAR SYSTEM

Complications
• Contractures
• Decreased muscle tone
• Muscle atrophy
Nursing interventions
• Turn and position your patient regularly, as needed.
• Make sure his body's properly aligned, and that his joints and muscles are well supported.
• Perform range-of-motion (ROM) exercises at least three times a day.
• Use supportive devices, as needed, such as footdrop stops, splints, trochanter rolls, and hand-rolls.
• When possible, reduce edema by elevating extremities.
• Hyperextend your patient's hips at least three times daily.

GASTROINTESTINAL SYSTEM

Complications
• Anorexia
• Ileal stasis
• Distention
• Diarrhea
• Constipation

Continued

Dealing with Daily-Care Complications
Continued

GASTROINTESTINAL SYSTEM
Continued

• Stress ulcers
Nursing interventions
• Make sure your patient has a high-roughage, balanced diet, with many of his food preferences.
• Arrange for your patient to have several small meals throughout the day instead of three large ones.
• Encourage adequate fluid intake; provide your patient with 1,000 to 2,000 ml of fluid daily, unless contraindicated.
• Check patient's abdomen every 4 hours for bowel sounds and distention. If distention occurs, measure patient's abdomen every 4 to 8 hours as ordered, and notify the doctor.
• Monitor bowel habits. Note amount, color, and consistency of stools.
• Check your patient's bowel-movement history. If he's constipated, make sure his medication isn't the cause.
• Administer stool softeners, as needed.
• For defecation, place your patient in a sitting position, if possible.
• Provide privacy for your patient when he's defecating.
• As soon as the patient's physi-

cal and neurologic condition allows, gradually increase his activities.
• Connect nasogastric tube to intermittent, low suction for 24 to 48 hours; then to gravity for 24 hours.
• If feeding via nasogastric tube, make sure feedings are easily digestible and high in protein.
• If patient can't tolerate feedings, notify doctor. He may order total parenteral nutrition.
• Maintain accurate intake and output records.
• Observe for signs and symptoms of stress ulcers, especially in patients receiving high doses of corticosteroids.
• Administer antacids and cimetidine (Tagamet*) prophylactically, if ordered.

GENITOURINARY SYSTEM

Complications
• Urinary retention
• Renal calculi
• Urinary tract infections
Nursing interventions
• Observe your patient's abdomen for bladder distention. If you suspect distention, palpate the area to confirm your findings, and notify the doctor.

NEUROLOGIC INJURIES

*Available in both the U.S. and Canada.

Continued

Dealing with Daily-Care Complications
Continued

GENITOURINARY SYSTEM
Continued

• Check urine for sediment, which may indicate early formation of renal calculi. If you note any sediment, send a specimen to the lab for analysis. Document the results, and notify the doctor if necessary.
• Minimize formation of new renal calculi by acidifying your patient's urine. Make sure he gets adequate amounts of vitamin C. Encourage him to drink orange or cranberry juice, or administer urine acidifiers, as ordered.
• Provide at least 1,500 to 2,000 ml of fluids daily, unless contraindicated.
• To prevent infection, change indwelling (Foley) catheter routinely; provide catheter care; and avoid irrigations.
• Administer urinary tract germicides, such as methenamine mandelate (Mandelamine*), as ordered.
• Don't give your patient foods that leave an alkaline ash residue in his urine, such as tomato juice.
• When your female patient needs to urinate, place her in a sitting position to allow good urine drainage. If your patient's a male and he's able, have him stand with assistance alongside the bed. Also, provide privacy.

• Turn and position patient every 2 hours, or as ordered.
• Perform complete range-of-motion (ROM) exercises at least three times a day.

SKELETAL SYSTEM

Complications
• Backaches
• Osteoporosis of disuse (intense pain with weight bearing)
• Contractures
Nursing interventions
• To prevent hip and knee flexion, turn and position your patient regularly, according to his needs.
• Make sure his body's properly aligned and that his joints and muscles are well supported.
• Help patient perform complete ROM and isometric exercises, as ordered, at least three times a day. Establish a daily program of resistive muscle exercises.
• Encourage mobility, and weight bearing, if not contraindicated. Periodically, try to stand your patient upright so he bears his weight, or use a tilt table.
• Be sure footboards are used properly. Place your patient's feet flat against the footboard so they form a 90° angle to his legs.
• Be sure patient's mattress is firm. Use a bedboard if necessary.

*Available in both the U.S. and Canada.

NEUROLOGIC INJURIES

Continued

Dealing with Daily-Care Complications
Continued

SKELETAL SYSTEM
Continued

• Make sure your patient gets a high-protein, low-calcium diet with plenty of fluids.
• Check his urine for sediment, which may indicate early formation of renal calculi. If you note any sediment, send a urine specimen to the lab for analysis. Document the results and notify the doctor, if necessary.
• To prevent constipation, provide a high-roughage diet; administer stool softeners; give plenty of fluids; establish good bowel routine; and be sure patient's well supported in sitting position during defecation, if possible.

CARDIOVASCULAR SYSTEM

Complications
• Decreased myocardial tone
• Venous stasis
• Thrombus formation
• Orthostatic hypotension
Nursing interventions
• To alleviate signs and symptoms of orthostatic hypotension, gradually elevate head of bed to sitting position, dangle his legs over side of bed prior to chair sitting, and stand patient before placing him in chair.
• To prevent increased workload on the patient's heart, instruct him how to turn with minimal effort, use overhead frame with trapeze bar, and take deep, slow breaths while turning.
• Gradually increase your patient's activities to avoid fatigue.
• Apply antiembolism stockings, as ordered. Remove them at least once every 24 hours.
• Elevate legs at hips rather than knees. Keep legs elevated above heart level.
• Place a pillow between patient's legs while he's on his side. Keep his upper leg positioned more anteriorly than his lower leg.
• Encourage foot and leg exercises.
• Make sure your patient has a high-protein, low-calcium diet, with plenty of fluids.
• Instruct your patient to exhale slowly when moving in bed to prevent him from performing a Valsalva maneuver.

NEUROLOGIC INJURIES

Combating the Effects of Immobility with Exercise

Regardless of your patient's neurologic disorder, you'll be responsible for helping plan and implement an exercise program tailored to his condition and needs. An effective exercise program, performed at least three times a day, will help your patient function at maximum capacity during his hospital stay and at home.

When we talk about an exercise program, we're referring to range-of-motion (ROM) exercises that take your patient's joints through their full extent of movement. These exercises also maintain joint activity, stimulate blood circulation, and promote muscle tone.

Where do you begin? First, you'll need to check your patient's care plan, medical history, physical condition, and emotional status. Consult with your patient's doctor and physical therapist. Depending on your hospital's policy, they may select your patient's ROM exercise program, or instruct you to do so.

The three basic types of ROM programs are:
● Active: helps strengthen weakened joints and is performed by the patient.
● Active-assistive: helps strengthen and maintain joint activity and motion. The patient performs these exercises with minimal assistance form another person.
● Passive: maintains joint activity and motion. These exercises are performed for the patient by another person; for example, a nurse or family member.

Before beginning your patient's exercise program, explain its importance to your patient and his family. Answer any questions they may have. Encourage the patient to be as active as physically possible. Also take this opportunity to encourage the family to take part in the patient's exercise program. Besides physically helping the patient (if needed), remind them that they play an important part in supporting and encouraging the patient. Then, show the patient and his family the complete program.

Document the procedure, program selected, and any patient teaching, in your nurses' notes.

Anticonvulsants

ACETAZOLAMIDE

375 mg to 1 g P.O. daily in divided doses

Interactions
Ephedrine, pseudoephedrine: increased CNS stimulation
Lithium: decreased therapeutic effects
Methenamine: antagonized methenamine effect

Side effects
Aplastic anemia, hyperchloremic acidosis

Special considerations
Obtain CBC and serum electrolytes every 3 months. Also, drug is usually given with other anticonvulsants. Monitor for hyperglycemia in prediabetics or diabetics on insulin or oral drugs.

CARBAMAZEPINE

800 mg to 1.2 g P.O. daily in divided doses

Interactions
Nicotinic acid: may decrease carbamazepine levels. Monitor for lack of therapeutic effect.
Propoxyphene: may increase carbamazepine levels. Use another analgesic.
Troleandomycin, erythromycin, isoniazid: may increase carbamazepine blood levels. Use together cautiously.

Side effects
Blood dyscrasias, dizziness, drowsiness, ataxia, nausea, stomatitis, dry mouth

Special considerations
May cause mild-to-moderate dizziness when first taken. Effect usually disappears within 4 days. Obtain CBC and platelet counts weekly for first 3 months, then monthly. Tell patient to notify doctor immediately if fever, sore throat, mouth ulcers, or easy bruising occurs. When used for trigeminal neuralgia, an attempt should be made every 3 months to decrease dose or to stop drug.

CLONAZEPAM

0.5 to 2 mg P.O. t.i.d.

Interactions
None significant.

Side effects
Drowsiness, ataxia, increased salivation

Special considerations
Warn patient to avoid activities that require alertness and good psychomotor coordination until CNS response to drug has been determined. Never withdraw drug suddenly. Tell patient to report side effects immediately. Also monitor patient for oversedation.
Continued

NEUROLOGIC DRUGS

Anticonvulsants
Continued

DIAZEPAM

For status epilepticus: 5 to 20 mg by slow I.V. push; may repeat q 5 to 10 minutes to maximum dose of 60 mg
Interactions
None significant
Side effects
Cardiovascular collapse, drowsiness, ataxia, pain at injection site, thrombophlebitis
Special considerations
Don't mix with other drugs or I.V. fluids. Avoid storing in plastic syringe or infusing through plastic tubing. Infuse at rate not exceeding 5 mg/minute and preferably at 2 mg/minute to decrease risk of respiratory depression and hypotension. Monitor respirations every 5 to 15 minutes and before each repeated dose. Have emergency resuscitative equipment and oxygen at bedside. Also watch for phlebitis at injection site.

ETHOSUXIMIDE

20 mg/kg P.O. in divided doses; maximum dose—1.5 g daily
Interactions
None significant
Side effects
Nausea, vomiting, anorexia, epigastric distress, drowsiness, euphoria, dizziness, blood dyscrasias

Special considerations
Warn patient to avoid activities that require alertness and good psychomotor coordination until CNS response to drug has been determined. Obtain CBC every 3 months. Never withdraw drug suddenly.

ETHOTOIN

2 to 3 g P.O. daily in divided doses
Interactions
Alcohol, folic acid, loxapine: decreased ethotoin activity
Oral anticoagulants, antihistamines, chloramphenicol, diazepam, diazoxide, disulfiram, isoniazid, phenylbutazone, salicylates, valproate: increased ethotoin activity and toxicity
Side effects
Nausea, vomiting, diarrhea, lymphadenopathy
Special considerations
Give after meals. Schedule doses as evenly as possible over 24 hours. Stop drug at once if lymphadenopathy or lupus-like syndrome develops. Hydantoin derivative of choice in young adults who are prone to gingival hyperplasia caused by phenytoin. Otherwise, it's infrequently used for treating epilepsy.

Continued

Anticonvulsants
Continued

MEPHENYTOIN

200 to 600 mg P.O. daily in three divided doses
Interactions
Alcohol, folic acid, loxapine: decreased mephenytoin activity
Oral anticoagulants, antihistamines, chloramphenicol, diazepam, diazoxide, disulfiram, isoniazid, phenylbutazone, salicylates, valproate: increased mephenytoin activity and toxicity
Side effects
Drowsiness, blood dyscrasias, skin rash, exfoliative dermatitis
Special considerations
Tell patient to notify doctor if fever, sore throat, bleeding, or skin rash occurs. These signs may indicate serious blood dyscrasias. Check CBC and platelet count initially and every 2 weeks thereafter, up to 2 weeks after full dose attained; then monthly. Stop drug if neutrophil count falls below 1,600/mm³.

MEPHOBARBITAL

Interactions
MAO inhibitors: potentiates barbiturate effect
Oral anticoagulants: possible decreased anticoagulant effect
Rifampin: may decrease barbiturate levels. Monitor for decreased effect.

Side effects
Dizziness, drowsiness, lethargy, skin eruptions
Special considerations
Warn patient to avoid activities that require alertness and good psychomotor coordination until CNS response to drug has been determined. Store drug in light-resistant container. In adults, give total or largest dose at night if seizures occur then. Warn patient to use drug cautiously with alcohol, narcotics, or other CNS depressant.

PARALDEHYDE

For status epilepticus: 5 to 10 ml I.M.; 0.2 to 0.4 ml/kg in 0.9% saline by I.V. injection
Interactions
Alcohol: increased CNS depression. Use together cautiously.
Disulfiram: increased paraldehyde blood levels; possible toxic disulfiram reaction. Use together cautiously.
Side effects
Pulmonary edema or hemorrhage, circulatory collapse (from I.V. use), foul breath odor, skin rash
Special considerations
Divide 10 ml I.M. dose into two injections. Inject deeply, away from

NEUROLOGIC DRUGS

Continued

Anticonvulsants
Continued

PARALDEHYDE
Continued

nerve trunks, and massage injection site. Use glass syringe and bottle for parenteral dose since drug reacts with plastic. Don't use if solution is brown or has a vinegary odor, or if container has been open longer than 24 hours.

PARAMETHADIONE

0.9 to 2.4 g P.O. daily in three or four divided doses
Interactions
None significant
Side effects
Blood dyscrasias, drowsiness, exfoliative dermatitis, skin rash, photophobia
Special considerations
Tell patient to immediately report sore throat, fever, malaise, bruises, petechiae, or epistaxis. Advise him to wear dark glasses if photophobia occurs.

PHENOBARBITAL

For status epilepticus: 10 mg/kg by I.V. infusion no faster than 50 mg/minute; maximum dose—20 mg/kg
For epilepsy: usual maintenance dose—100 to 200 mg P.O. daily in single or divided doses
Interactions

Alcohol and other CNS depressants, including narcotic analgesics: excessive CNS depression.
MAO inhibitors: potentiated barbiturate effect.
Oral anticoagulants: possible decreased antiocoagulant effect.
Rifampin: may decrease barbiturate levels. Monitor for decreased effect.
Side effects
Lethargy, drowsiness, hangover, skin eruptions
Special considerations
Reserve I.V. injection for emergency treatment, and give slowly under close supervision. Monitor respirations carefully. Watch for signs of barbiturate toxicity: asthmatic breathing, cyanosis, clammy skin, hypotension, coma. Overdose can be fatal.

Don't use injection solution if it contains a precipitate.

PHENSUXIMIDE

500 mg to 1 g P.O. b.i.d. or t.i.d.
Interactions
None significant
Side effects
Nausea, vomiting, drowsiness, dizziness
Special considerations
Never withdraw drug suddenly to avoid petit mal seizures. Report side effects immediately. Drug may cause pink, red, or reddish-brown urine. *Continued*

Anticonvulsants
Continued

PHENYTOIN

For status epilepticus: 500 mg to
1 g I.V. at 50 mg/minute
For epilepsy: maintenance dose—
300 to 600 mg P.O. daily or in divided doses
Interactions
Alcohol, folic acid, loxapine: decreased phenytoin activity
*Oral anticoagulants, antihista-
mines, chloramphenicol, cimetidine, diazepam, diazoxide,
disulfiram, isoniazid, phenylbutazone, salicylates, thioridazine, valproate:* phenytoin toxicity risk
Side effects
Nausea, vomiting, gingival hyperplasia, blood dyscrasias, rash, exfoliative dermatitis, hirsutism,
nystagmus, diplopia, blurred vision, drowsiness, dizziness, confusion, hallucinations, slurred
speech
Special considerations
Give divided doses with or after
meals to decrease GI side effects.
Stop drug if skin rash appears. If
rash is scarlet or measles-like, resume drug after rash clears. If
rash reappears, stop drug. If rash
is exfoliative, purpuric, or bullous,
don't resume drug. Provide patient with instructions.
  Use only clear solution for injection. Consider slight yellowing
acceptable. Don't refrigerate drug.

PRIMIDONE

250 mg P.O. t.i.d. or q.i.d.
Interactions
Carbamazepine: increased primidone levels. Observe for toxicity.
Phenytoin: stimulates conversion of
primidone to phenobarbital. Observe for increased phenobarbital
effect.
Side effects
Drowsiness, diplopia, lethargy,
nausea, vomiting
Special considerations
Warn patient to avoid activities that
require alertness and good psychomotor coordination until CNS response to drug has been determined. Drug is partially converted to
phenobarbital by body metabolism.
Shake liquid suspension well.

VALPROIC ACID, VALPROATE SODIUM

15 to 30 mg/kg daily, usually in divided doses
Interactions
Antacids, aspirin: may cause valproic acid toxicity. Use together
cautiously and monitor blood levels.
Side effects
Nausea, vomiting, indigestion,
thrombocytopenia, hepatotoxicity

Continued

Anticonvulsants
Continued

VALPROIC ACID, VALPROATE
SODIUM
Continued

Special considerations
Obtain liver function studies, platelet counts, and prothrombin time before starting drug and every month thereafter. Nonspecific symptoms, such as fever and lethargy, may signal severe hepatotoxicity.

Anti-infectives

CEFOTAXIME

---

1 g I.V. or I.M. q 6 to 8 hours; maximum dose—12 g daily in life-threatening infections
Interactions
Probenecid: may inhibit excretion and increase blood levels of cefotaxime
Side effects
Diarrhea, pseudomembranous colitis, rash, urticaria, pain at injection site, thrombophlebitis (with I.V. administration)
Special considerations
Give drug I.V. rather than I.M. in life-threatening infection. When administering I.M., inject deep into a large muscle mass, such as the gluteus or lateral aspect of thigh.

CHLORAMPHENICOL

---

50 to 100 mg/kg P.O. or I.V. daily in divided doses q 6 hours; maximum dose—100 mg/kg daily
Interactions
Acetaminophen: elevated chloramphenicol levels
Oral anticoagulants: possible bleeding
Penicillins: antagonized antibacterial effect. Give penicillin at least 1 hour before.
Sulfonylureas: increased hypoglycemia
Side effects
Aplastic anemia, granulocytopenia, dose-related anemia
Special considerations
Monitor CBC, platelet and reticulocyte counts, and serum iron levels before and every 2 days during therapy. Stop drug immediately if anemia, reticulocytopenia, leukopenia, or thrombocytopenia develops.

Continued

Anti-infectives
Continued

MOXALACTAM

2 to 6 g I.V. or I.M. daily in divided doses q 8 hours; maximum dose —12 g daily in life-threatening infections
Interactions
Ethyl alcohol: may cause disulfiram-like reaction. Warn patient not to drink alcohol for several days after discontinuing moxalactam.
Side effects
Hypoprothrombinemia with possible severe bleeding, diarrhea, pseudomembranous colitis, rash, urticaria, pain at injection site, thrombophlebitis
Special considerations
When administering I.M., inject deep into a large muscle mass, such as the gluteus or lateral aspect of thigh. If severe bleeding occurs after high doses, promptly give vitamin K.

NAFCILLIN

2 to 12 g I.V. or I.M. daily in divided doses q 4 to 6 hours
Interactions
Aminoglycoside antibiotics: separate I.V. nafcillin dose by at least 1 hour. Don't mix together in same I.V. container.
Chloramphenicol, erythromycin, *tetracyclines:* antibiotic antagonism. Give nafcillin at least 1 hour before.
Probenecid: increased blood levels of nafcillin. (Probenecid is often used for this purpose.)
Side effects
Hypersensitivity, skin rash, thrombophlebitis
Special considerations
Before giving nafcillin, ask patient if he's had any allergic reactions to penicillin. Check drug's expiration date. Give intermittently I.V. to prevent vein irritation. Also change site every 48 hours.

VIDARABINE

15 mg/kg daily for 10 days; give by slow I.V. infusion over 12 to 24 hours
Interactions
Allopurinol: increased incidence of CNS side effects
Side effects
Anorexia, nausea, tremor, dizziness, confusion
Special considerations
Don't give I.M. or S.C. because of low solubility and poor absorption. Administer with an in-line I.V. filter 0.45 μm or smaller. CNS side effects must be distinguished from symptoms of encephalitis.

NEUROLOGIC DRUGS

Antimyasthenics

NEOSTIGMINE

15 to 30 mg P.O. t.i.d.; 0.5 to 2 mg I.M. or I.V. q 1 to 3 hours, as needed

Interactions

Procainamide, aminoglycoside antibiotics, quinidine: may reverse cholinergic effect on muscle. Observe for lack of therapeutic effect.

Succinylcholine: prolonged respiratory depression and possible apnea

Side effects

Nausea, vomiting, diarrhea, muscle cramps, respiratory depression

Special considerations

Monitor vital signs frequently, especially respirations. Keep atropine injection available to treat serious side effects. Give drug with milk or food to reduce GI side effects. Document patient's response after each dose. Show patient how to observe and record variations in muscle strength.

PYRIDOSTIGMINE

60 to 180 mg P.O. b.i.d. or q.i.d. with maximum dose of 1,500 mg; 2 mg I.M. or very slow I.V. injection q 3 hours

Interactions

Procainamide, aminoglycoside antibiotics, quinidine: may reverse cholinergic effect on muscle. Observe for lack of therapeutic effect.

Succinylcholine: prolonged respiratory depression and possible apnea

Side effects

Nausea, vomiting, diarrhea, headache

Special considerations

Parenteral dose is $\frac{1}{30}$ of oral dose. Double-check all orders for I.M. or I.V. administration. Adjust dose depending on patient response.

Antineoplastics

CARMUSTINE (BCNU)

100 mg/m² by slow I.V. infusion daily for 2 days; repeat dose q 6 weeks if platelets above 100,000/mm³ and WBC above 4,000/mm³

Interactions

Cimetidine: increased bone marrow suppression. Avoid use if possible.

Side effects

Bone marrow suppression, including leukopenia and thrombocytopenia; nausea; vomiting; pain at infusion site; pulmonary fibrosis

Continued

Antineoplastics
Continued

CARMUSTINE (BCNU)
Continued

Special considerations
Warn patient to watch for signs of infection and bone marrow suppression, such as fever, sore throat, anemia, fatigue, easy bruising, nose or gum bleeds, and tarry stools. Take temperature daily. To reduce pain on infusion, dilute drug further or slow the infusion rate. Avoid contact with skin, as carmustine causes a brown stain. If drug comes into contact with skin, wash off thoroughly. Solution is unstable in plastic I.V. bags. Administer only in glass containers.

LOMUSTINE (CCNU)

130 mg/m^2 P.O. in a single dose q 6 weeks; give only if platelets above 100,000/mm^3 and WBC above 4,000/mm^3
Interactions
None significant
Side effects
Bone marrow suppression, including leukopenia and thrombocytopenia; nausea; vomiting
Special considerations
Give drug 2 to 4 hours after meals. To avoid nausea, give antiemetic before administering. Monitor blood counts weekly. Don't give more often than every 7 weeks; bone marrow suppression is cumulative and delayed.

Antiparkinson Drugs

LEVODOPA

0.5 to 1 g P.O. daily b.i.d., t.i.d., or q.i.d. Increase dose by 0.75 g every 3 to 7 days; maximum dose— 8 g daily
Interactions
Antacids: may increase levodopa effect
Anticholinergic drugs, tricyclic antidepressants, benzodiazepines, clonidine, papaverine, phenothiazines and other antipsychotics, *phenytoin:* decreased levodopa effect
Pyridoxine: decreased levodopa effect. Check vitamin preparations and nutritional supplements for content of vitamin B$_6$ (pyridoxine).
Side effects
Choreiform, dystonic and dyskinetic movements; involuntary grimacing; myoclonic body jerks; psychiatric disturbances; nausea; vomiting; anorexia; orthostatic hypotension

Continued

Antiparkinson Drugs
Continued

LEVODOPA
Continued

Special considerations
Adjust dose according to patient's response. Monitor vital signs, especially while adjusting dose. Warn patient of possible dizziness and orthostatic hypotension, especially at start of therapy. Inform patient and family that multivitamin preparations, fortified cereals, and certain over-the-counter drugs may contain pyridoxine (vitamin B_6), which can reverse the effects of levodopa.

LEVODOPA-CARBIDOPA

3 to 6 tablets of 25 mg carbidopa/250 mg levodopa P.O. daily in divided doses; maximum dose—8

tablets daily
Interactions
Papaverine, diazepam, clonidine, phenothiazines and other antipsychotics: may antagonize Parkinsonian actions. Use together cautiously.
Side effects
Choreiform, dystonic, and dyskinetic movements; involuntary grimacing; myoclonic body jerks; orthostatic hypotension
Special considerations
Adjust dose according to patient's response. Drug effects occur more rapidly with levodopa-carbidopa than with levodopa alone. Monitor vital signs, especially while adjusting dose. If patient is receiving levodopa, discontinue this drug for at least 8 hours before starting levodopa-carbidopa.

Antithrombotics

ASPIRIN

1,300 mg P.O. daily
Interactions
Ammonium chloride (and other urine acidifiers): increased aspirin levels. Monitor for aspirin toxicity.
Antacids in high doses (and other urine alkalinizers), corticosteroids:

decreased aspirin effect.
Oral anticoagulants and heparin: increased risk of bleeding.
Side effects
Prolonged bleeding time, nausea, vomiting, GI distress, and occult bleeding
Special considerations
Advise patients receiving large
Continued

Antithrombotics
Continued

ASPIRIN
Continued

doses of aspirin for an extended period to watch for petachiae, bleeding gums, and GI bleeding, and to maintain adequate fluid intake. Give with food, milk, antacid, or water to reduce GI side effects. Obtain hemoglobin levels and prothrombin time periodically.

DIPYRIDAMOLE

For transient ischemic attacks:
400 to 800 mg P.O. daily in divided doses
Interactions
None significant
Side effects
Headache, dizziness, hypotension, nausea
Special considerations
Give 1 hour before meals. Monitor blood pressure and observe for side effects, especially with large doses. Also watch for signs of bleeding and for prolonged bleeding time.

HEPARIN

7,500 to 10,000 units by I.V. bolus, then 1,000 units hourly by I.V. infusion

Interactions
Aspirin: may increase bleeding risk. Don't use together.
Side effects
Hemorrhage and excessive bleeding, thrombocytopenia
Special considerations
Measure partial thromboplastin time (PTT) carefully and regularly. Anticoagulation exists when PTT values are 1.5 to 2 times control values.

When intermittent I.V. therapy is used, always draw blood 30 minutes before next scheduled dose to avoid spuriously elevated PTT.

Avoid excessive I.M. injections of other drugs to prevent or minimize hematomas.

SULFINPYRAZONE

For transient ischemic attacks:
600 to 800 mg P.O. daily in divided doses
Interactions
Oral anticoagulants: possible bleeding
Probenecid: inhibited renal excretion of sulfinpyrazone. Use together cautiously.
Side effects
Nausea, dyspepsia, epigastric pain
Special considerations
Give with milk, food, or antacid to reduce GI side effects.

Continued

NEUROLOGIC DRUGS

Antithrombotics
Continued

WARFARIN

Maintenance dose—2 to 10 mg daily P.O.

Interactions
Allopurinol, chloramphenicol, danazol, clofibrate, diflunisal, dextrothyroxine, thyroid drugs, heparin, anabolic steroids, cimetidine, disulfiram, glucagon, inhalation anesthetics, metronidazole, quinidine, influenza vaccine, sulindac, sulfonamides: increased prothrombin time. Monitor for bleeding.

Ethacrynic acid, indomethacin, mefenamic acid, oxyphenbutazone, phenylbutazone, salicylates: increased prothrombin time; ulcerogenic effects.

Griseofulvin, haloperidol, carbamazepine, paraldehyde, rifampin: reduced anticoagulant effect.

Glutethimide, chloral hydrate, sulfinpyrazone, triclofos sodium: increased or decreased prothrombin time.

Side effects
Hemorrhage and excessive bleeding, dermatitis, skin rash, fever

Special considerations
Regularly measure prothrombin time (PT) to monitor anticoagulant effect. PT should be 1.5 to 2 times normal. When PT exceeds 2.5 times control value, bleeding risk is high.

Give drug at the same time daily. Stress importance of complying with recommended dose and keeping follow-up appointments. Advise patient to carry a card that identifies him as a potential bleeder. Also suggest that he use an electric razor when shaving to avoid scratching skin and to brush his teeth with a soft toothbrush. Tell female patient to report unusually heavy menses. The dose may need to be adjusted.

Fever and skin rash signal severe complications. Elderly patients and those with renal or hepatic failure are especially sensitive to warfarin effect.

Heavy Metal Antagonists

DIMERCAPROL

2 to 5 mg/kg by deep I.M. injection daily to q.i.d.

Interactions
131I uptake thyroid tests: decreased iodine uptake. Don't schedule patient for this test during course of dimercaprol therapy.
Iron: formed toxic metal complex. Don't use together.

Side effects
Transient hypertension, tachycardia, nausea, vomiting, renal damage

Special considerations
Give only by deep I.M. route, and massage injection site after giving drug. Drug has an unpleasant, garlicky odor.

Keep urine alkaline to prevent renal damage. Oral NaHCO₃ may be ordered.

EDETATE CALCIUM DISODIUM

1 g in 500 ml of 5% dextrose of 0.9% sodium chloride by I.V. infusion; 1 g I.M.

Interactions
None significant

Side effects
Nephrotoxicity with acute tubular necrosis, fever, and chills 4 to 8 hours after infusion

Special considerations
Encourage fluids to promote excretion of edetate-metal complex (except in lead poisoning, since excess fluid may raise ICP). Monitor intake and output, urinalysis, BUN, and EKGs. To avoid toxicity, use drug with dimercaprol. Procaine HCl may be added to I.M. solutions to minimize pain. Avoid rapid I.V. infusions, and watch for local reactions afterward.

Miscellaneous Drugs

DEXAMETHASONE

For cerebral edema: 10 mg I.V., then 4 to 6 mg I.M. q 6 hours for 2 to 4 days; then decrease dose over 5 to 7 days

Interactions
Indomethacin, aspirin: increased risk of GI distress and bleeding. Use together cautiously.

Continued

Miscellaneous Drugs
Continued

DEXAMETHASONE
Continued

Side effects
Atrophy at I.M. injection sites, euphoria, insomnia, peptic ulcer

Special considerations
Give I.M. injection deep into gluteal muscle. Avoid S.C. injections, which may result in atrophy and sterile abscesses. When possible, replace I.M. with P.O. route.

DISULFIRAM

For chronic alcoholism: 125 to 500 mg P.O. daily

Interactions
Alcohol: disulfiram reaction (blurred vision, confusion, dyspnea, tachycardia, hypotension, flushing, nausea, vomiting, sweating, thirst, vertigo).
Isoniazid (INH): ataxia or marked change in behavior. Avoid use.
Metronidazole: psychotic reaction. Don't use together.
Paraldehyde: toxic levels of the acetaldehyde. Don't use together.

Side effects
Drowsiness, headache, garlic-like taste, peripheral neuritis

Special considerations
Warn patient to avoid all alcohol, including that found in foods, medications, and toiletries. Tell him that disulfiram reaction may occur as long as 2 weeks after

single dose of disulfiram. The longer patient remains on drug, the more sensitive he becomes to alcohol. Blood alcohol level of 5 to 10 mg/dl may trigger a mild reaction; a level of 50 mg/dl a severe reaction; unconsciousness usually occurs at level of 125 to 150 ml/dl. Reaction may last ½ hour to several hours, or as long as alcohol remains in blood. Reassure patient that most side effects subside after 2 weeks of therapy.

ERGOTAMINE

For migraine headache: 2 mg P.O. or S.L., then 1 to 2 mg P.O. hourly or S.L. q ½ hour. Maximum dose—6 mg daily

Interactions
Beta-adrenergic blockers: possible increased vasoconstriction

Side effects
Numbness and tingling in fingers and toes, muscle pains

Special considerations
Most effective when used during prodromal stage of headache or as soon as possible after onset. Sublingual tablet is preferred during early stage of attack because of its rapid absorption. Prolonged exposure to cold weather should be avoided whenever possible. Cold may increase side effects. Avoid prolonged use and don't exceed recommended dosage.
Continued

Miscellaneous Drugs
Continued

LACTULOSE

For hepatic coma: 20 to 30 g (30 to 45 ml) P.O. t.i.d. or q.i.d. until patient has two or three soft stools daily
Interactions
None significant
Side effects
Cramps, belching, flatulence, diarrhea, hypernatremia
Special considerations
If desired, minimize drug's sweet taste by diluting with water or fruit juice or giving with food. Reduce dosage if diarrhea occurs. Replace fluid loss. Monitor serum sodium for possible hypernatremia, especially with high doses.

METHYSERGIDE

For migraine headache prophylaxis: 2 to 4 mg P.O. b.i.d. with meals
Interactions
None significant
Side effects
Retroperitoneal and pulmonary fibrosis, vertigo, euphoria
Special considerations
Stop drug every 6 months; then restart after at least 3 or 4 weeks. Tell patient not to stop drug abruptly; may cause rebound headaches. Stop gradually over 2 to 3 weeks. Not for treatment of migraine or vascular headache in progress.

NEOMYCIN

For hepatic coma: 1 to 3 g P.O. q.i.d. for 5 to 6 days
Interactions
Dimenhydrinate: may mask symptoms of ototoxicity
Ethacrynic acid, furosemide: increased ototoxicity
Other aminoglycosides, methoxyflurane: increased ototoxicity and nephrotoxicity
Side effects
Ototoxicity, nephrotoxicity
Special considerations
Drug isn't absorbed at recommended dosage. However, more than 4 g of neomycin daily may be systemically absorbed and may lead to nephrotoxicity. Monitor renal function (urine output, specific gravity, BUN and creatinine levels, and creatinine clearance). Notify doctor of signs of decreasing renal function.

PROPRANOLOL

For migraine headache prophylaxis: 160 to 240 mg P.O. daily in divided doses or once daily as sustained-release capsule
Interactions
Barbiturates, rifampin: decreased effect of propranolol.
Chlorpromazine, cimetidine: increased effect of propranolol.

Continued

Miscellaneous Drugs
Continued

PROPRANOLOL
Continued

Insulin, oral hypoglycemics: monitor patient for altered dosage requirements.
Side effects
Fatigue, lethargy, bradycardia, heart failure, heart block, hypotension
Special considerations
Monitor blood pressure for hypo-tension due to propranolol's beta-blocking action. To improve poor compliance with therapy, change dosage schedule to once or twice daily. Recognize that drug masks common signs of shock and hypoglycemia. Drug is for prophylaxis only; it won't effectively treat migraine already in progress.

Controlling Seizures with Phenytoin

Dear Patient,
Your doctor has prescribed phenytoin (Dilantin) to help you control seizures. Remember:
• Carry identification saying that you use this drug. Report its use before any surgery or emergency treatment.
• Take phenytoin exactly as your doctor orders, preferably at the same time(s) each day.
• Tell your doctor immediately if you're pregnant, nursing, or planning a pregnancy; if you have or develop any other medical conditions; or if you're taking any other prescription or nonprescription drugs.
• Don't start or stop taking any other drugs without first asking your doctor. Any change may alter phenytoin's effectiveness.
• If you're taking *liquid phenytoin*, shake the bottle well and use a medical measuring spoon to ensure correct dosage. If you're taking *phenytoin tablets*, chew or crush them. If you're taking *capsules*, swallow them whole.

Continued

Controlling Seizures with Phenytoin
Continued

• If phenytoin upsets your stomach, ask your doctor about taking it with food or milk. Also ask about use of alcohol, which may alter the drug's effectiveness.

• Miss a dose? *If you normally take one dose a day,* take the missed dose immediately, then resume your normal schedule. However, if you don't remember the missed dose until the next day, don't take it and don't double your daily dose; just resume your normal schedule. *If you normally take several doses a day,* take the missed dose immediately (unless your next scheduled dose is within 4 hours), then resume your normal schedule. Don't double-dose. *If you miss doses for 2 or more days,* call your doctor.

• See your doctor regularly, especially at first, since your dosage may need adjusting.

• Don't stop taking this drug without first asking your doctor. Abrupt withdrawal may cause adverse reactions.

• Call your doctor immediately if you develop involuntary eye movements, blurred or double vision, skin rash, drowsiness, dizziness, confusion, hallucinations, slurred speech, or other adverse reactions.

• Don't be alarmed if phenytoin causes gray stool and pink to reddish-brown urine.

• Because phenytoin may cause gum tenderness, swelling, or bleeding, brush and floss carefully and see your dentist regularly.

• When refilling your prescription, don't change brands or dosage forms or allow generic substitutions without first asking your doctor. Phenytoin comes in several forms, and each acts differently in the body.

Anticonvulsant Medications

PHENOBARBITAL
(Luminal*)

Usual dose
5 to 10 mg/kg/day in children
Indications
Grand mal, focal seizures, psychomotor seizures
Toxic signs
Nystagmus, ataxia
Side effects
Sedation, megaloblastic anemia

PHENYTOIN SODIUM
(Dilantin*)

Usual dose
5 to 10 mg/kg/day in children
Indications
Grand mal, focal seizures
Toxic signs
Nystagmus, ataxia, lethargy
Side effects
Gum hyperplasia, megaloblastic anemia

PRIMIDONE
(Mysoline*)

Usual dose
10 to 20 mg/kg/day in children
Indications
Grand mal, focal seizures, psychomotor seizures
Toxic signs
Ataxia, nystagmus, lethargy
Side effects
Sedation, nausea and vomiting

TRIMETHADIONE (Tridione*)

Usual dose
300 mg/2 to 3 times a day in children
Indications
Petit mal
Toxic signs
Sedation, nausea
Side effects
Acneiform rash, aplastic anemia, blurred vision

ETHOSUXIMIDE (Zarontin*)

Usual dose
250 mg twice a day in children
Indications
Petit mal
Toxic signs
Dizziness, nausea and vomiting
Side effects
Rash, leukopenia

CLONAZEPAM
(Clonopin, Rivotril*)

Usual dose
0.1 to 0.2 mg/kg/day maintenance dose in children
Indications
Petit mal, myoclonic seizures
Toxic signs
Ataxia, hypersalivation, drowsiness
Side effects
Behavior changes

*Also available in Canada

Comparing Anticonvulsants

DRUG	BLOOD LEVELS (mcg/ml)	HALF-LIFE	TIME TO REACH STEADY STATE*
carbamaze-pine	6 to 8	7 to 30 hr	2 to 4 days
clonazepam	0.013 to 0.072	20 to 30 hr	5 to 10 days
ethosuxim-ide	40 to 80	2 to 3 days	5 to 8 days
methsuxim-ide	0.1	2 to 4 hr	8 to 16 hr
phenobarbi-tal	10 to 35	2 to 4 days	14 to 21 days
phenytoin	10 to 20	24 hr	5 to 10 days
primidone	6 to 12	3 to 12 hr	4 to 7 days
trimetha-dione	6 to 41	12 to 24 hr	2 to 5 days
valproic acid	50 to 100	5 to 20 hr	2 to 4 days

*Steady-state blood levels are achieved if the patient is initially given maintenance therapy rather than a loading dose.

Use of Anticonvulsants in Epileptic-Type Seizures

DRUG	GENERALIZED TONIC-CLONIC (GRAND MAL)	ABSENCE (PETIT MAL)
Barbiturate derivatives		
mephobarbital	✔	✔
metharbital	✔	✔
phenobarbital	✔	✔
primidone	✔	
Benzodiazepine derivatives		
clonazepam		✔
diazepam		
Hydantoin derivatives		
ethotoin	✔	
mephenytoin	✔	
phenacemide		
phenytoin	✔	

MYOCLONIC	MIXED	COMPLEX-PARTIAL (PSYCHO-MOTOR)	STATUS EPILEPTICUS
✔	✔		
✔	✔	✔	
		✔	
✔			
			✔
		✔	
		✔	
	✔	✔	
		✔	✔

Continued

NEUROLOGIC DRUGS

Use of Anticonvulsants in Epileptic-Type Seizures
Continued

DRUG	GENERALIZED TONIC-CLONIC (GRAND MAL)	ABSENCE (PETIT MAL)
Oxazolidone derivatives		
paramethadione		✔
trimethadione		✔
Succinimide derivatives		
ethosuximide		✔
methsuximide		✔
phensuximide		✔
Miscellaneous		
acetazolamide		✔
bromides*	✔	✔
carbamazepine	✔	
valproic acid		✔

MYOCLONIC	MIXED	COMPLEX-PARTIAL (PSYCHOMOTOR)	STATUS EPILEPTICUS
✔	✔	✔	
	✔	✔	

*Rarely used as drug of first or second choice
Note: Magnesium sulfate and paraldehyde are not included in this list since they are used to control nonepileptic seizures.

Corticosteroid

DEXAMETHASONE (Decadron*)

Indications and dosage
Cerebral edema
Adults: Initially, 10 mg (phosphate) I.V. then 4 to 6 mg I.V. or I.M. every 6 hours for 2 to 4 days; then decrease dosage over 5 to 7 days.
Inflammatory conditions, allergic reactions, neoplasia
Adults: 0.25 to 4 mg P.O. b.i.d., t.i.d., or q.i.d. or 4 to 16 mg (acetate) I.M. into joint or soft tissue every 1 to 3 weeks; or 0.8 to 1.6 mg (acetate) into lesions every 1 to 3 weeks.

Side effects
Euphoria; insomnia; psychotic behavior; congenital heart failure; hypertension; edema; cataracts; glaucoma; increased intraocular pressure; peptic ulcer; GI irritation; increased appetite; severe hypokalemia; hyperglycemia; carbohydrate intolerance; glycosuria; impaired wound healing; various skin eruptions, including acne; muscle weakness; pancreatitis; hirsutism; and susceptibility to infections. Acute adrenal insufficiency may follow increased stress (such as infection, surgery, trauma) or abrupt withdrawal after long-term therapy.
Note: Most side effects of corticosteroids are dose- or duration-related.

*Available in both the U.S. and Canada.

Withdrawal symptoms: rebound inflammation; fatigue; weakness; arthralgia; fever; dizziness; lethargy; depression; fainting; orthostatic hypotension; dyspnea; anorexia; and hypoglycemia

Interactions
• Barbiturates, phenytoin sodium (Dilantin*), and rifampin (Rifadin*) cause *decreased* corticosteroid effect.
• Indomethacin (Indocin), and aspirin (A.S.A.): cause *increased risk* of GI distress and bleeding. Administer dexamethasone (Decadron*) cautiously when patient is also receiving indomethacin (Indocin) and aspirin (A.S.A.).

Precautions
• Contraindicated in systemic fungal infections, and for alternate-day therapy.
• Use cautiously in GI ulceration or renal disease: hypertension; osteoporosis; varicella; vaccinia; exanthem; diabetes mellitus; Cushing's syndrome; thromboembolic disorders; seizures; myasthenia gravis; metastatic cancer; congestive heart failure; tuberculosis; ocular herpes simplex; hypoalbuminemia; and emotional instability or psychotic tendencies.
• *Sudden withdrawal may be fatal.*

Continued

Corticosteroid
Continued

DEXAMETHASONE
Continued

Nursing considerations
• Give I.M. injection deep into gluteal muscle. Avoid subcutaneous administration, as atrophy and sterile abscesses may occur.
• Monitor patient's weight, blood pressure, and serum electrolyte and serum glucose levels.
• Inspect patient's skin for petechiae. Warn patient that he will bruise easily.

• Instruct patient to carry a card indicating his need for supplemental systemic glucocorticoids during stress, especially as dose is decreased.
• Tell patient not to discontinue drug abruptly without doctor's consent.
• Teach patient signs of early adrenal insufficiency; for example, fatigue, muscle weakness, and joint pain.

Diuretic

MANNITOL (Osmitrol*)

Indications and dosage
Edema.
100 g as a 10% to 20% solution over 2 to 6 hour period.
To reduce intraocular pressure or intracranial pressure (ICP).
1.5 to 2 g/kg as a 20% to 25% solution I.V. over 30 to 60 minutes.

Side effects
Rebound increase in ICP 8 to 12 hours after diuresis; transient expansion of plasma volume during infusion, causing circulatory overload and pulmonary edema; headache; confusion; tachycardia; angina-like chest pain; blurred vision; rhinitis; thirst; nausea; vomiting; urinary retention; fluid and electrolyte imbalances; water intoxication; cellular dehydration

Interactions
None significant

Precautions
• Contraindicated in anuria; severe pulmonary congestion; pulmonary edema; severe congestive heart disease; severe
Continued

*Available in both the U.S. and Canada.

Diuretic
Continued

MANNITOL
Continued

dehydration; metabolic edema; progressive renal disease or dysfunction; progressive heart failure during administration; active intracranial bleeding, except during craniotomy.

Nursing considerations
• Monitor vital signs, including central venous pressure (CVP), and intake/output, hourly (report increasing oliguria).
• Monitor daily weights, renal function, fluid balance, and serum electrolytes including serum osmolality level.

• During diuretic therapy to reduce intracranial pressure, alternate drug with furosemide (Lasix*), as ordered.
• Administer infusions I.V. via an in-line filter.
• Solution may crystallize, especially at low temperatures. To redissolve, warm bottle in hot water bath, and shake it vigorously. Cool to body temperature before administering. Do not use solution with undissolved crystals.
• Give frequent mouth care or fluids to relieve thirst.
• Observe I.V. site for signs and symptoms of infiltration, such as: inflammation, edema, and potential necrosis.

Histamine Receptor Antagonist

CIMETIDINE (Tagamet*)

Indications and dosage
Duodenal ulcer prophylaxis
Adults and children over 16 years: 300 mg I.V. or P.O. every 6 hours. Maximum daily dose is 2,400 mg.
Side effects
Confusion; dizziness; mild and transient diarrhea; perforation of chronic peptic ulcers after abrupt

cessation of drug; interstitial nephritis; transient elevations in blood urea nitrogen (BUN) and serum creatinine levels; jaundice; acne-like rash; urticaria; exfoliative dermatitis; hypersensitivity; muscle pain; reduced sperm count; mild gynecomastia after use longer than 1 month (but with no change in endocrine function).

Continued

*Available in both U.S. and Canada.

NEUROLOGIC DRUGS

Histamine Receptor Antagonist
Continued

CIMETIDINE
Continued

Interactions
• Antacids may interfere with drug absorption. Allow 1 hour between administration of cimetidine (Tagamet*) and antacids.
• Warfarin-type anticoagulants potentiated by cimetidine (Tagamet*). Monitor prothrombin time closely.
• Antimetabolites and alkylating agents administered with drug will cause a decrease in white blood cells, and agranulocytosis.
Precautions
• Elderly patients are more susceptible to cimetidine-induced confusion. Doses should be decreased in elderly patients and in patients with renal insufficiency.
• Symptomatic response to drug therapy does not rule out possibility of a malignant gastric tumor.
• Large parenteral doses should be avoided in asthmatic patients.
Nursing considerations
• I.M. route of administration is contraindicated.
• Administer with meals to maintain blood levels.
• Hemodialysis reduces blood level of cimetidine (Tagamet*). Schedule cimetidine dose at end of hemodialysis treatment.
• I.V. solutions compatible for dilution are: normal saline solution, 5% and 10% dextrose (and combinations of these), lactated Ringer's solution and 5% sodium bicarbonate injection.
• Do not dilute medication with sterile water for injection.
• Slightly elevated serum creatinine levels may be observed.

Analgesic
Narcotic

CODEINE (sulfate, phosphate)

Indications and dosage
Mild to moderate pain
Adults: 15 to 60 mg P.O. or 15 to 60 mg (phosphate) subcutaneous or I.M. every 4 hours, as needed.
Side effects
Sedation; clouded sensorium; euphoria; convulsions (with large doses); hypotension, bradycardia; nausea; vomiting; constipation; ileus; urinary retention; respiratory depression; physical dependence
Interactions
General anesthetics; other narcotic analgesics; tranquilizers; sedatives; hypnotics; alcohol; tricyclic antidepressants; MAO inhibitors

*Available in both U.S. and Canada.

NEUROLOGIC DRUGS

Continued

Analgesic
Continued

CODEINE
Continued

Precautions
Use with extreme caution in patients with head injuries; increased intracranial pressure; increased cerebrospinal fluid pressure; severe central nervous system depression; respiratory depression; hepatic or renal disease; hypothyroidism; Addison's disease; acute alcoholism; seizures; chronic obstructive pulmonary disease (COPD); shock; or in elderly or debilitated patients.
Nursing considerations
• Use cautiously—analgesics will

cause increased central nervous system (CNS) depression.
• For full analgesic effect, give before patient has intense pain.
• To potentiate effect of codeine sulfate, administer with aspirin (A.S.A.) or acetaminophen (Tylenol*).
• Do not administer discolored injection solution.
• Monitor respiratory and circulatory status, including urine output and bowel function.
• Instruct ambulatory patients that codeine sulfate causes drowsiness, and they should avoid activities that require alertness and good psychomotor coordination, such as driving a vehicle.

Analgesic
Nonnarcotic, antipyretic

ACETAMINOPHEN (Tylenol*)

Indications and dosage
Mild pain or fever
Adults and children over 10 years: 325 to 600 mg P.O. or rectally every 4 hours, as needed. Maximum 2.6 g daily.
Side effects
Severe liver toxicosis with massive doses; rash; urticaria
Interactions
None significant

*Available in both U.S. and Canada.

Precautions
High doses or unsupervised chronic use can cause liver damage. Excessive ingestion of alcoholic beverages may enhance liver toxicosis.
Nursing considerations
Administer acetaminophen (Tylenol*) to patients allergic to or unable to tolerate aspirin (A.S.A.). *Note:* acetaminophen has no anti-inflammatory effect.

NEUROLOGIC DRUGS

Guide to Some Drugs that Affect the Nervous System

CLASSIFICATION	POSSIBLE SIDE EFFECTS
Adrenergic blockers (sympath-olytics) methysergide maleate (Sansert*)	• Vertigo, light-headedness, insomnia, drowsiness, ataxia, hyperesthesia, euphoria, hallucinations
Aminoglycosides All types	• Neuromuscular blockage, headache, lethargy
Anticonvulsants phenytoin sodium (Dilantin Sodium*)	• Headache, ataxia, slurred speech, insomnia, lethargy
Antidepressants amitriptyline hydrochloride (Elavil*) phenelzine sulfate (Nardil*)	• Headache, drowsiness, confusion, tremors
Antihypertensives hydralazine hydrochloride (Apresoline*) methyldopa (Aldomet*)	• Headache, dizziness
Antipsychotics All types	• Extrapyramidal reactions
Antituberculars, antileprotics ethambutol hydrochloride (Myambutol*)	• Headache, dizziness, confusion, peripheral neuritis

NEUROLOGIC DRUGS

Continued

*Available in both U.S. and Canada. **Available in Canada only. All other products (no symbol) are available in the U.S. only.*

Guide to Some Drugs that Affect the Nervous System
Continued

CLASSIFICATION	POSSIBLE SIDE EFFECTS
Antituberculars, antileprotics *Continued* streptomycin sulfate	• Transient paresthesias, especially circumoral
Cerebral stimulants All types	• Headache, dizziness, insomnia, tremor, hyperactivity
Cholinergics physostigmine salicylate (Antilirium*)	• Restlessness, twitching, ataxia, sweating
Corticosteroids All types	• Pseudotumor cerebri
Gastrointestinal agents metoclopramide hydrochloride (Reglan**)	• Headache, dizziness, restlessness, drowsiness
Nonnarcotic analgesics and antipyretics indomethacin (Indocin)	• Headache, dizziness, drowsiness, confusion, peripheral neuropathy, convulsions
Psychotherapeutics lithium salts (Lithane*)	• Headache, dizziness, drowsiness, restlessness, tremors, confusion, lethargy, ataxia, epileptiform seizures, blackouts

NEUROLOGIC DRUGS

Continued

Guide to Some Drugs that Affect the Nervous System
Continued

CLASSIFICATION	POSSIBLE SIDE EFFECTS
Spasmolytics theophylline salts (Elixophyllin*)	• Headache, dizziness, restlessness, insomnia, convulsions
Tetracyclines doxycycline hyclate (Vibramycin*) oxytetracycline hydrochloride (Terramycin*)	• Benign intracranial hypertension, dizziness
Urinary tract germicides nitrofurantoin (Furadantin)	• Headache, dizziness, peripheral neuropathy, drowsiness
Vinca alkaloids vinblastine sulfate (Velban) vincristine sulfate (Oncovin*)	• Loss of deep tendon reflex, numbness, paresthesias, peripheral neuropathy and neuritis
Miscellaneous chloramphenicol (Chloromycetin*)	• Headache, confusion, peripheral neuropathy with prolonged therapy
levodopa (Levopa*)	• Nervousness, fatigue, malaise, choreiform and dystonic movements, psychiatric disturbances, ataxia

*Available in U.S. and Canada. **Available in Canada only. All other products (no symbol) are available in the U.S. only.

NEUROLOGIC DRUGS

INDEX

INDEX

INDEX

INDEX

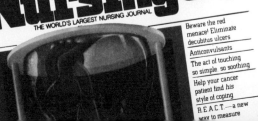